thefacts

Depression

E

➔ also available in the**facts** series

ADHD, SECOND EDITION
Selikowitz
978-0-19-956503-0 | July 2009

Alcoholism, FOURTH EDITION
Manzardo
978-0-19-923139-3 | July 2008

Alzheimer's and other Dementias
Hughes
978-0-19-959655-3 | August 2011

Angina and Heart Attack
Jevon
978-0-19-959928-8 | November 2011

Breast Cancer
Saunders
978-0-19-955869-8 | June 2009

COPD
Currie
978-0-19-956368-5 | March 2009

Cosmetic Surgery
Waterhouse
978-0-19-921882-0 | March 2008

Depression, SECOND EDITION
Wasserman
978-0-19-960293-3 | October 2011

Down Syndrome, THIRD EDITION
Selikowitz
978-0-19-923277-2 | May 2008

Epilepsy, THIRD EDITION
Appleton
978-0-19-923368-7 | January 2009

Heart Disease
Chenzbraun
978-0-19-958281-5 | August 2010

Insomnia and Other Adult Sleep Problems
Stores
978-0-19-956083-7 | January 2009

Lung Cancer, THIRD EDITION
Falk
978-0-19-956933-5 | October 2009

Obsessive-Compulsive Disorder, FOURTH EDITION
Rachman
978-0-19-956177-3 | March 2009

Osteoporosis
Black
978-0-19-921589-8 | February 2009

Panic Disorder, THIRD EDITION
Rachman
978-0-19-957469-8 | October 2009

Post-traumatic Stress
Regel
978-0-19-956658-7 | April 2010

Pre-Natal Tests and Ultrasound
Burton
978-0-19-959930-1 | September 2011

Prostate Cancer, SECOND EDITION
Mason
978-0-19-957393-6 | June 2010

Pulmonary Arterial Hypertension
Handler
978-0-19-958292-1 | June 2010

Schizophrenia, THIRD EDITION
Tsuang
978-0-19-960091-5 | August 2011

Sexually Transmitted Infections, THIRD EDITION
Barlow
978-0-19-959565-5 | March 2011

Sleep Problems in Children and Adolescents
Stores
978-0-19-929614-9 | November 2008

The Pill and Other Forms of Hormonal Contraception, SEVENTH EDITION
Guillebaud
978-0-19-956576-4 | July 2009

the**facts**

Depression
SECOND EDITION
DANUTA WASSERMAN

Professor in Psychiatry and Suicidology,
Head of the Swedish National Prevention of Suicide
and Mental Ill-Health (NASP) at Karolinska Institute,
Stockholm, Sweden, and Director of the WHO Leading
Collaborating Centre on Mental Health and
Prevention of Suicide, Copenhagen,
Denmark, and Geneva, Switzerland

OXFORD
UNIVERSITY PRESS

OXFORD

UNIVERSITY PRESS

Great Clarendon Street, Oxford OX2 6DP

Oxford University Press is a department of the University of Oxford.
It furthers the University's objective of excellence in research, scholarship,
and education by publishing worldwide in

Oxford New York

Auckland Cape Town Dar es Salaam Hong Kong Karachi
Kuala Lumpur Madrid Melbourne Mexico City Nairobi
New Delhi Shanghai Taipei Toronto

With offices in

Argentina Austria Brazil Chile Czech Republic France Greece
Guatemala Hungary Italy Japan Poland Portugal Singapore
South Korea Switzerland Thailand Turkey Ukraine Vietnam

Oxford is a registered trade mark of Oxford University Press
in the UK and in certain other countries

Published in the United States
by Oxford University Press Inc., New York

© Oxford University Press, 2011

British Library Cataloguing in Publication Data

Data available

Library of Congress Cataloging in Publication Data

Data available

ISBN 978-0-19-960293-3

10 9 8 7 6 5 4 3 2

Typeset in Plantin by Cenveo, Bangalore, India
Printed in Great Britain
on acid-free paper by
Ashford Colour Press Ltd, Gosport, Hampshire

Preface

Depression is a broad term, involving a spectrum that ranges from mild despondency to melancholia, the very deepest form of depression. Natural despondency is not a disease but simply a part of life. Perhaps it may even be the case that we need down periods and the occasional blues to develop, mature, and form our personality. Depression, however, is a psychiatric illness that must be identified and treated in the same manner as other illnesses.

Many famous writers, musicians, artists, politicians, and scientists have occasionally been deeply depressed. Today it is known that depression as a mental illness is much more common than earlier believed, but also there are effective treatment methods that help. No one should have to suffer unnecessarily.

With the background of my experiences as professor and psychiatrist at the Karolinska Institute, I saw that there was a need for a general and elementary book in which the perspectives of both the natural and social sciences were brought to bear on the subject of depression. This book draws on the knowledge gained from extensive research within both biological and psychosocial fields.

I would like to thank my husband, Professor Jerzy Wasserman, who not only encouraged me to write it, but also actively contributed with a review of the current literature in the leading scientific journals. I have also taken advantage of criticism after our long discussions where both the biological and psychological aspects have been treated.

It is my hope that this book shall be of particular interest to the general reader, sufferers, and their friends and families, and that it will be of support and help to those that need it.

Danuta Wasserman,

Stockholm, Sweden 2011

Contents

List of abbreviations   ix

PART 1
Symptoms of depression

1 Sorrow and natural despondency   3

2 Mood disorders   11

3 Seasonal depressions   21

4 Depression in childhood and adolescence   25

5 Women, men, and depression   35

6 The elderly and depression   43

7 Physical illness, pain, symptoms, and depression   49

8 Substance abuse and depression   55

9 Eating disturbances and depression   59

10 Anxiety and depression   63

11 Sleep and depression   69

PART 2
Causes of depression

12 Biological theories on the causes of depression   77

13 Psychological theories of depression   81

14 Nature or nurture: what matters most?   85

PART 3
Treatment of depression

15 When to see a doctor and subsequent treatment   91

16 Treatment with antidepressant medication   99

17 Sexuality, depression, and antidepressant medication   105

18 Electroconvulsive therapy and light therapy   109

19 Psychological forms of treatment   115

20 Advice to family members   125

21 Self-help in depression   131

22 Suicide and depression: when zest for life is gone   137

Index   147

List of abbreviations

BLT	bright-light therapy
CBT	cognitive behavioural therapy
CT	cognitive therapy
DBT	dialectic behavioural therapy
ECT	electroconvulsive treatment
GAD	generalized anxiety disorder
HRT	hormone replacement therapy
IPT	interpersonal psychotherapy
MAO	monoamine oxidase
MS	multiple sclerosis
OCD	obsessive–compulsive disorders
PPD	postpartum depression
PTSD	post-traumatic stress disorder
REM	rapid eye movement
RIMA	reversible inhibitor of MAO-A
SAD	seasonal affective mood disorder
SNRI	serotonin and noradrenaline reuptake inhibitors
SSRI	selective serotonin reuptake inhibitors
TCA	tricyclic antidepressants
TMS	transcranial magnetic stimulation

PART 1

Symptoms of depression

1

Sorrow and natural despondency

 Key points

- Feeling low or despondent can be natural at certain stages of life that are exciting, stressful and trying.

- Crises vary in intensity depending on the situation—short-term depression following a crisis is normal.

- Grief can last for 6 months or longer and can manifest itself in physical and psychological symptoms.

- The intensity of bereavement depends on the individual previous experiences, social network, and culture.

- Half of those who grieve or feel despondent show one or more symptoms of depression such as: insomnia, tearfulness, or lack of appetite.

- Talking about the grief, sorrow, dejection, irritation, and anger we experience is vital for our mental and physical wellbeing.

- 'Adjustment disorder' (a prolonged stress reaction) is when uncomplicated grief gives way to prolonged emotional or behavioural disturbances.

We all go through the natural periods of sorrow and despondency in life. Despondency can indicate that we should slow down, rest, reflect, and try to change negative situations.

We may succumb to sadness and dejection in response to trying situations in life, such as: death, divorce, unemployment, bankruptcy, war, or terrorist attacks. Men's grief and sorrow is often expressed in behavioural changes, and in some cases aggression; whereas in women sadness and dejection can be seen. Despondency can have an important survival function, resulting in reorientation and maturation.

Transitional phases

> How would it be, my dear,
> If grief one day came near,
> Filled your life
> With pain and strife,
> And emptied it of cheer?
> No need to answer now—
> I was just wondering how.
>
> Translated from Nils Ferlin, Swedish Poet (1898–1961)

No one can expect to always feel positive and happy. On some mornings one wakes up full of energy; on others staying in bed seems preferable. This is entirely normal. Feeling low or despondent is natural especially when we bid farewell to one stage of life and face the task of finding new paths. At the crossroads, people commonly ask themselves questions, such as: What is the purpose of my life? What shall I concentrate on? How important is it to do what I'm about to do? What is the worst thing that can happen?

Life stages and paths which may trigger despondency can include:

- Leaving the parental home

- Choice of partner

- Reaching the mid-years (30–40 years old)

- Menopause

- Unemployment

- Retirement.

Tribulations

Tribulations such as dismissal, work overload, bankruptcy, divorce, illness, and exile, affect a growing number of people. Crises vary in intensity depending on the type of loss, previous experiences, and present situation. Whether the crisis turns into depression depends upon personality. Support, from family or colleagues, also has a bearing on whether depression emerges.

Dejection and depression in response to existential crises have tangible causes and do not need any medical or psychological treatment. As a crisis is such a universal phenomenon, we can obtain help from each other's experiences and find workable solutions. However, this is possible only if we acknowledge our changed life situation and are prepared to tackle it. This is why daring to admit and talk about the grief, sorrow, dejection, irritation, and anger we experience is so important.

If the crisis culminates in resolution of a conflict or brings about some essential change in a person's life it can serve a positive purpose. The same may be said of natural despondency and of depression. However, it is vital for a person who feels depressed and whose normal way of life is hampered by mental and other symptoms to seek professional help.

Bereavement

> Everything I ever owned
> Belonged to you more than to me.
> Everything I wanted most
> Was yours, all yours to be.
> Life itself is dead and gone
> Now you are here no more.
> The world's a vast and empty shell,
> An apple with no core.
>
> Translated from Karin Boye, Swedish Poet (1901–41)

The intensity and duration of grief depends upon personality, previous experience, cultural factors, social networks, and the type of loss. This is why its symptoms and course are different for each person. Some forms of grief never really go away, although we can live a normal life. Memories and recollections may crop up at any time, and they almost invariably do on anniversaries and remembrance days.

Feelings of loss and grief might be for:

+ A lost child or beloved spouse

+ A country lost owing to war or exile

+ Relatives or friends lost through genocide.

Some people grieve for 6 months, others for perhaps a year or even longer. In normal grief we experience not only psychological pain but physical manifestations which diminish over time. These might include:

+ Palpitations

+ Stomach cramps

+ A lump in the throat

+ Tension aches in the head, neck, or jaw

- Disturbed dreams

- Hallucinations about a person or place

- Crying.

Profound grief very often arouses unease and fear in others, even in the nearest and dearest relatives and friends of the bereaved. One of the most common ways of reacting to sorrow is crying, which is an important way of expressing despair and pain and has a healing effect. Mourning entails many feelings besides sorrow and dejection. Mourners may be bitter about their situation or the deceased, and feel as if they have been let down. Irritation and anger are other common feelings connected with the disappointment of being left behind and abandoned.

Adjustment disorder: a prolonged stress reaction

Sleepless she lay,
Counting the four squares
Of moonlight on the floor.
When she rose and went to the window,
Over the meadows she saw the moon,
And fear, loneliness, the lunar path,
Unrest and sorrow filled her soul.

Translated from Harry Martinson, Swedish writer and
Nobel Prize Laureate (1904–78)

Half of all those who grieve, feel sad and despondent, and show one or more symptoms of depression such as insomnia and poor appetite. These reactions do not usually require treatment. In certain cases, on the other hand, grief, crises, bereavement, or severe trauma may become more complicated and lead to 'adjustment disorder' and depression. This may occur if, for example, the person concerned has been heavily dependent on, or had a complicated relationship with, the deceased. Where such relationships accommodated both love and hate, their sudden interruption due to death may cause the survivors to experience intense guilt and anger.

Prolonged stress reaction (also called adjustment disorder) is diagnosed when uncomplicated grief gives way to emotional or behavioural disturbances owing to further stress and strains in life.

Common symptoms of adjustment disorder are:

- Despondency

- A sense of hopelessness

◆ Tearfulness

◆ Inability to cope

◆ Anguish.

This diagnosis is made if the reaction is disproportionately strong or unusually long. Normally, symptoms do not last longer than 6 months, and usually disappear when the person's life situation changes or the stressor ceases. In chronic states, symptoms may last more than 6 months, partly owing to the persistence of the stressful life event or its consequences.

Treatment for adjustment disorder

Most people have the capacity to recover unaided from a severe crisis, grief, or a stressful situation. However, sometimes we cannot cope, or do not feel strong enough to deal with such matters. We should not suffer unnecessarily, and each of us must decide for ourselves whether we need professional help. The perception of pain is subjective. What one person can cope with may overwhelm another. The lines between grief, natural despondency, and depression are highly individual.

📄 Sophie, aged 59: adjustment disorder with depressed mood

Three years ago, Sophie was widowed. After 30 happy years with her beloved Albert, he died suddenly from a heart attack. For some time, Sophie had seen Albert's health deteriorating; he had been tired, suffered from marked dizziness, and felt weak. Albert had often complained of chest pains, radiating towards his jaw and the pit of his stomach. When Albert arrived at the hospital after collapsing at work, he was found to be having an acute heart attack. He was immediately admitted to an intensive-care unit. A few days later, he had another heart attack. This time, he did not survive.

When Sophie returned to the house that evening, she broke down. She cried and was utterly beside herself. She ran up and down the stairs, screaming in desperation. Although exhausted, she steeled herself to arrange the funeral and make all the other practical arrangements. She did not want anyone's help.

Their only child, a son who had lived and worked in Australia for several years, returned home for the funeral but had to go back straight after it. He had his work and family to think about. After the funeral Sophie isolated herself. She disconnected the telephone. She did not want to talk to or see anyone. Instead, she sat and stared at portraits of Albert. The days passed. She cried, slept little, ate from time to time, and did nothing in particular. Sometimes it felt as if Albert was just away temporarily. She lost count of time.

In the year after Albert's death, Sophie imagined that Albert was returning to her in the form of a bird that used to land on the windowsill. She fantasized that Albert was coming to tell her that he was fine, and wanted to see how she was getting on after his death. She talked about her sorrows and everyday problems. The conversation with Albert in the bird's guise felt very real to her, although at the same time she knew it was just a fantasy. When Sophie eventually went to see a doctor, she told him about her conversations with Albert. The doctor prescribed no medication, but she continued to visit him regularly.

After this period of extreme despair, which lasted nearly 2 years, Sophie began to feel angry. She was angry with Albert for leaving her, not looking after his heart properly, and putting her in this difficult situation. The anger gave her energy, and she decided to sell the house. She found a flat and put energy into renovating it. She accepted invitations from relatives to take part in family occasions and spend weekends with them. Eventually she was again able to speak of Albert with tenderness, and expressed gratitude for the love she had been able to experience.

Three years after Albert's death, the acute grief she felt subsided, giving way to a sense of loss. Sophie still works, and sometimes travels to see relatives. She has also taken up her previous hobbies. The memory of Albert remains strong; she thinks of him every day.

George, aged 50: grief

I suppose I've never really been depressed. Sometimes I've felt sad, such as when a business deal fell through. I was also sad when Christopher, my eldest son, broke off his studies and decided to become an artist. Sometimes I wonder how things would be today if he'd taken over my firm in Texas (USA).

But when my father died, everything happened so fast. By the time I realized he was dying, it was already too late to talk to him. There was so much unsaid between us. When my father divorced my mother, I was 18. I was furious with him for many years. Then he remarried, and there was always something that stopped me from talking to him.

After the funeral I felt really bad. I couldn't sleep at night, and sometimes I had a cry. I wouldn't have believed it of myself. Somehow it felt better after I'd cried, but I was ashamed as well. I took a week off work to get away to our holiday cottage. There I found myself talking to my dead father and wondering why we'd never got closer to each other. In spite of everything, he was a decent man. During that week I often went to see John, a farmer who helps us with our holiday cottage. We talked about everything, and suddenly it just came up how I felt when my father, whom I enjoyed being with so much, divorced my mother. That helped.

Although I felt so bad after my father's death, I knew somehow that it would pass. It's natural to feel like that when a close relative dies. John, who listened to me, had also opened his door so that I could see what his life was like. And he, too, seemed grateful to get a chance of talking about the kinds of things that felt hard to bear. It was as if my grief helped me to discover John's problems, and other people's as well. I think I've got better at recognizing when people are sad or don't feel good, even if they keep quiet about it. Nowadays it feels natural for me to ask my employees how they feel and whether there's anything they'd like to talk about. Previously, I would never have dreamt of intruding on other people with questions like that.

2

Mood disorders

➲ Key points

◆ The main types of depression are: major depression and persistent depression (dysthymia).

◆ The characteristics of major depression are: despondency, low spirits, inability to feel joy, appetite changes, sleep problems and fatigue, low self-esteem, concentration problems, and thoughts about death.

◆ Melancholia is a severe form of major depression when one is low-spirited with an inability to shift the heavy, dark mood. This is an illness that cannot be altered by external stimuli.

◆ Persistent depression or dysthymia is when despondency has been shown for at least 1–2 years alongside problems with appetite, sleep, lack of energy, self-esteem, concentration, and feelings of hopelessness. Symptoms can however be diverted by external stimuli.

◆ Double depression is when a dysthymic also suffers from major depression.

◆ Manic-depressive illness, also called 'bipolar disorder', is character-ized by extreme mood swings. A person's mood oscillates between deep depression and elation known as mania.

Depression, like manic-depressive illness, belongs to a group of illnesses relating to the emotions. In medical science they are known as the 'affective disorders', and their onset is often subtle with no obvious external cause. The duration and severity of depression varies.

At dawn,
when the dream-struck coin of night
turns over,
and ribs, skin, eyeballs
are sucked into their own birth—
the white-crested cockerel crows,
the terrible moment of godless penury has come
and a crossroads reached—
Madness is the monarch's drummer—
blood, becalmed, is shed—

> Translated from Nelly Sachs, German-Jewish poet,
> Living in Sweden and Nobel Prize Laureate (1891–1970)

How a diagnosis is reached

The typical sadness and natural despondency we experience in conjunction with various events (such as death of a loved one) count as a natural reaction, not a mental illness. Sometimes, however, people have a very strong psychological reaction to difficulties in life, traumatic experiences, crises, and catastrophes. This is different from depression and is known as 'adjustment disorder' (also termed 'prolonged stress reaction') which may be accompanied by despondency and anguish (Figure 2.1). The stress reaction may be acute or, if it lasts more than 6 months, become chronic.

There are two main types of depression: major depression, and persistent depression (dysthymia). Just under half of depressed patients succumb to depression once in their lives, the remaining half often suffer from relapses, i.e. become depressed again after being entirely or partially free from symptoms. There is, unfortunately, one type of depression—chronic depression—in which the sufferer never really becomes entirely well between depressive episodes.

Major depression

Children, young people, adults, and the elderly alike can be afflicted. The most common symptoms of major depression are:

- **Despondency:** Low spirits for most of the day, virtually every day.

- **Anhedonia (joylessness):** Reduced interest and pleasure in most activities.

- **Appetite changes:** Loss of appetite and weight; sometimes weight gain.

- **Disturbed sleep or insomnia:** Difficulty in falling asleep, early waking, or too much sleep.

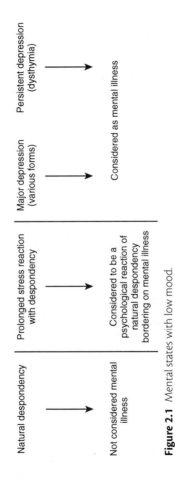

Figure 2.1 Mental states with low mood.

◆ **Change in motor activity:** Heavy, sluggish movements; reduced facial expressions; sometimes restlessness.

◆ **Fatigue:** Increased physical and mental tiredness.

◆ **Low self-esteem, sense of guilt:** Self-disparagement and unwarranted feelings of guilt.

◆ **Concentration difficulties:** Difficulties in concentrating, learning, and making decisions.

◆ **Thoughts about death and suicide, suicide attempts:** Recurrent thoughts about death, with persistent suicidal thoughts. Suicide plans or attempts.

In order for a major depression to be diagnosed at least five of the symptoms, always including despondency and anhedonia, must be observable. Moreover, the symptoms must be felt during the greater part of the day, and daily, for at least two weeks. The symptoms must impair work performance and social capacity. The diagnosis of major depression is not made if a person suffers from only a few symptoms for a short time.

When depression is diagnosed, one should take into consideration:

◆ The effect of the symptoms: their intensity and duration

◆ The course of the illness

◆ The incidence of previous depression

◆ Depression or manic-depressive illness in the family.

The most severe forms of major depression are melancholia and major depression with psychotic symptoms.

Melancholia

Typical psychological symptoms of melancholia are:

◆ Low, heavy spirits

◆ Being 'cheered up' merely feels painful

◆ Indifference to the outside world

◆ Being passive, withdrawn, and lacking energy

◆ Slow thinking and delayed reaction time

- Sluggish or lack of facial expressions

- Looking 10–15 years older than normal

- Self-belittlement and an exaggerated sense of guilt

- Feeling that life is pointless

- Feelings of failure in everything.

Physical symptoms characteristic of melancholia are:

- Marked decrease in appetite and weight loss

- Constipation

- Sexual disturbances

- Reduced tear and saliva excretion

- Insomnia.

Melancholics wake up early in the morning—roughly 2 or 3 hours earlier than normal. On waking, until the afternoon, they feel worried and anxious. Heavy spirits are unable to be diverted by external positive stimuli. The melancholic person can improve as the afternoon wears on. Sometimes, a sufferer may be free from symptoms in the evening and fall asleep normally, only to wake once more in the small hours, tormented by their symptoms and pronounced anguish.

Elizabeth, aged 58: major depression

Elizabeth's marriage is good. Her husband is kind and thoughtful, and they have a married daughter whom she gets on well with. For nearly 15 years, Elizabeth has battled against her demons. Life has very often felt arduous and grey, without any real reason. This is her own description of her illness:

'The first time I came into contact with the black hole inside me, I was 43 years old. I felt full of anxiety and low-spirited, without understanding why. Nothing in my life had changed. I slept badly, woke up before dawn, and lay there tossing and turning. I accused myself of all kinds of things, and brooded on the kind of mother I had been to my daughter. It felt as if I were the reason for the problems my husband had been having in relationships with his family. I believed that fate was going to punish us, and that something would happen to my daughter or my husband. It was difficult getting out of bed in the morning; some days, I didn't get up at all. I felt like a zombie, and hardly even managed to shower or wash my hair. When I saw my face in the mirror, it was like looking at a corpse. I was pale, washed-out, and looked rigid in some way. I ate nothing, although my husband tried to cook meals I liked. In a month, I lost nearly ten kilos.'

On that occasion, it took almost one year before the feelings of hopelessness and other symptoms abated. Then they reappeared when Elizabeth's daughter moved away to another town. Elizabeth slipped into a very deep pit of depression. When she went to see a doctor, he told her something that still rings in her ears: 'The illness you're suffering from is the easiest of all mental illnesses to cure. You won't die of it. It will pass.' He prescribed antidepressants, but Elizabeth broke off the treatment because the medication made her feel unwell. She tried another drug, but that did not suit her either. Her anguish became more and more acute, until it was almost unbearable. A doctor prescribed tranquillizers, and on one occasion she took 15–20 at once because she wanted to sleep. Hospitalized owing to this overdose, she received treatment.

'It was a relief, I was well looked after, and admitted to a psychiatric clinic. Before that, I hadn't fully realized the gravity of my situation.' Elizabeth was given a new type of antidepressant to try. Initially she felt sick and vomited, but the side-effects passed fairly rapidly. After she had suffered two more attacks of depression within a couple of years, the doctor prescribed long-term treatment. Today, Elizabeth is taking antidepressants continuously to prevent a new depression. She does not feel any particular side-effects, she is active once more, and her old anxiety is gone. 'I've got my life back.'

Major depression with psychotic symptoms

Alongside the depressive symptoms, depression with psychotic symptoms is characterized by a loss of capacity to grasp and relate to reality with the presence of delusions, cognitive disturbances, and visual or auditory hallucinations. Delusions in psychotic depression often have a depressive content caused by the person's life situation and mood.

Persistent depression (dysthymia)

Good morning, if it is a good morning . . .
Winnie the Pooh, in A.A. Milne, British writer (1882–1956)

The diagnosis of dysthymia is made if an adult shows despondency lasting at least 2 years combined with another two of the symptoms relating to appetite, sleep, lack of energy, self-disparagement, concentration difficulties, and feelings of hopelessness. For children and young people, it is enough for the symptoms to last at least 1 year. Symptoms such as irritability and impatience without despondency are characteristic of dysthymia in the young; this state is known as dysphoria.

Dysthymics very often talk about their unhappy childhood experiences and poor relationships with parents and siblings. Lack of self-esteem and relationship problems are also very common. Dysthymia is a form of depression that is intimately linked to the personality of the depressed individual. The dysthymic has a fundamentally depressive personality, with a pessimistic outlook on life. Even between the depressive episodes, dysthymics are gloomy and inhibited. This is in contrast to sufferers from major depression who have no obvious personality disorder.

Dysthymia, like major depression, occurs more often in women than in men. However, in contrast to severe major depression, such as melancholia, dysthymic symptoms can be diverted by external stimuli. This means that the despondency or irritation may lift if something enjoyable happens. However, the dysthymic's anxiety may be severe.

Amire, aged 48: dysthymia with episodes of major depression

Amire is an artist, married, with three adult children she gets on well with. She was born in Morocco, but has spent her entire adult life in France.

Since the age of 30, she has suffered from periods of despondency. There is a certain pattern to her typical day. On waking she feels slightly anxious, and this intensifies during the day. She worries about the present, the future, and her own health. These pronounced worries usually persist until late evening, when she feels worst of all. Amire very often has difficulty in falling asleep, although she is tired. After dropping off she sleeps poorly, wakes up after a few hours, and finds it difficult to get back to sleep.

During certain periods—which may come at any time of year—Amire feels markedly worse. Although she normally finds it agreeable to be alone, she is then tormented when her husband is not at home. She has difficulty in concentrating, and starts tasks she is incapable of completing. Lost in details, she cannot see the wood for the trees; this makes her irritated, and her own feeling is that it is impossible to try and talk her out of it. Amire is also disturbed by the slightest noise. She becomes upset when the telephone rings, and everyone has to tiptoe around her. She cannot stand light, and the blinds are often drawn. Owing to her tiredness she cannot cope with the cleaning, and the mess around her makes her even more overwrought and annoyed. She feels sorry for herself and close to tears, and thinks she will never be well again.

Amire also becomes physically run down during these periods and feels weak, although all medical examinations yield normal findings. As she constantly changes details in her paintings, she cannot complete any of her work. Several exhibitions have been postponed, and one was cancelled as she was dissatisfied with her work. Amire usually blames both herself and those closest to her for all the difficulties she is experiencing, and for her alleged failures in her profession. These accusations are not justified, as Amire's work is usually acclaimed and sought after.

Amire is plagued by a severe sense of guilt about her behaviour. When the depression abates, Amire enjoys running her home and looking after her family, but her existence is always characterized by gloom and uncertainty about her artistic achievements. She has been undergoing psychotherapy for several years. In the therapy, Amire has realized that she has a strong sense of abandonment; it has been there since her childhood, and she tries to fend it off in various ways. In the course of the therapy, childhood memories have surfaced. She recalls how she had difficulty in accepting her parents' tender feelings and how irritable she became when anyone praised her. She thought her parents were trying to humour her, to conceal what she perceived as their lack of love for her. But somewhere inside she knew that her parents loved and appreciated her.

Thanks to enhanced self-understanding. She feels less demanding of her husband, and thinks that their life together is better. Her old irritability, tearfulness, and constant tension have also released their hold. 'With the sun above and the earth below, we're growing together,' she says. Alongside the psychotherapy, Amire is taking antidepressants. She has learnt to cope with a few common side-effects, and the medication now suits her fairly well.

Manic-depressive illness

Manic-depressive illness, also called 'bipolar disorder', is characterized by mood swings. A person's mood may swing between deep depression and pathological elation known as mania. Between the depressive and manic episodes there are periods of complete or partial recovery. The number, duration, and severity of depressive and manic episodes vary from one person to the next. Some individuals experience depressive or manic episodes only a few times in their lives. For others, the intervals between periods of illness are short.

Characteristics of mania

Mania is characterized by a pathologically elated mood. A person in a manic phase has reduced sleep requirements, and a strong need to talk—often rapidly, incomprehensibly, and incoherently. Breaking off worthwhile connections with others, overestimating themselves, and exhibiting strikingly poor judgment are also characteristic features of manic people. They may appear impulsive, unpredictable, irritable, and easily provoked; sometimes, they become threatening and aggressive. Their frenetic and aimless activity may lead to social disasters, while ruined relationships may ensue from infidelity and disgrace. Heavy debts may be accrued as a result of impulse buying or ill-considered investments.

It is sometimes difficult for the closest relatives, and even experienced psychiatrists, to detect the initial signs of mania. People close to sufferers from hypomania (a milder form of mania) may sometimes become infected by the manic depressive person's optimism. At the beginning of an acute bout, a manic may be aware of the difference between normal and pathological and may give the impression of being entirely well.

Treatment of manic-depressive illnesses

It may take several years, with several episodes of illness, before a manic-depressive submits to the treatment programme required to keep the illness in check. Manic-depressive illness is treated successfully with mood-regulating drugs, such as lithium. Lithium treatment is often combined with psycho-therapy to help people cope with the social consequences of their illness. It is not unusual for manic or manic-depressive people to engage in 'self-medica-tion' with alcohol or drugs. Alcohol and drug abuse cause deterioration in the course of the illness and may trigger mania.

One important part of the treatment is for the patient to learn how to detect the early symptoms and contact a doctor to prevent the mania from develop-ing. If manic-depressive people learn to control their illness and comply with the treatment prescribed, they can live a good life.

For some people, hypomania seems to be an asset. It makes them creative, efficient, witty, and sociable. People with hypomanic characteristics often feel very good as a result of their hyperactivity, and get a great deal done. But this mild hypomanic phase can, in some people, rapidly give way to mania, especially in stressful situations.

Schizophrenia and depression

Schizophrenic people may become depressed as a result of their psychosocial life situation and the limitations imposed by their illness. Some medicines used to treat schizophrenia (so called neuroleptics) may cause depression. Schizophrenic and other psychotic people benefit if their treatment is com-bined with supportive psychotherapy and social rehabilitation. Providing sup-port for the schizophrenic's relatives and teaching them how to relate to the person without being either excessively protective or rejecting, is usually a valuable means of preventing adverse repercussions.

3

Seasonal depressions

➲ Key points

- ◆ Human beings are affected by rhythmic alternation between day and night, light and darkness, cold and warmth.

- ◆ Body temperature, digestion, secretion of hormones, and other physiological functions show a regular daily rhythm that follows the sleep cycle.

- ◆ Seasonal depression has some 'atypical' depressive symptoms such as increased sleep and appetite, especially cravings for carbohydrates.

- ◆ Winter depression is a type of despondency that returns year after year during the winter period. Its symptoms appear in the autumn, and abate in the spring when the hours of daylight increase.

- ◆ Women appear to be most susceptible to winter depression, and the symptoms usually appear between the ages of 20 and 30.

- ◆ Light therapy has proved highly effective in winter depression: as many as 80% of sufferers become entirely free from symptoms.

Major depression can be related to the seasons, where it recurs annually at the same time of year. In the northern hemisphere, people may become depressed by the November darkness which abates when the light returns in February or March. Seasonal depressions both in the southern and northern hemisphere have been associated with the onset of autumn/winter. Seasonal depression is also known as 'seasonal affective mood disorder' (SAD).

Body rhythms

I'm not angry with the spring—
that it's here again.
I don't blame it
for doing what it does every year:
its duty.

Translated from Wislawa Szymborska, Polish Poet,
Nobel Prize Laureate (b. 1923)

Like all other living organisms, human beings are affected by rhythmic alternation between day and night, light and darkness, cold and warmth. In the course of our evolution we have developed biological mechanisms to cope with these changes. Body temperatures, digestion, secretion of hormones, as well as various other physiological functions, show a regular daily rhythm that largely follows the wakefulness–sleep cycle. But in some of us these biological rhythms are subject to the seasons' influence more than in others.

For seasonal depression to be diagnosed there must be a recurrent chronological connection between the onset of depression and a particular time of year. This pattern must have occurred in at least two consecutive years. Alleviation of depression must also, as a rule, take place at the same time every year. People suffering from seasonally related depression show broadly the same clinical picture as people with major depression (see Chapter 2), except that they may show 'atypical' symptoms more frequently, such as increased sleep and appetite, especially cravings for carbohydrates.

Winter depression

Hippocrates, an ancient Greek physician and 'Father' of medicine (c. 460–377 BC) noted that some people adapt well and some poorly to the summer, and that the same applies to the winter. The most recognized form of seasonal affective disorder (SAD) known as 'winter depression' has attracted particular interest owing to the good results obtained from light therapy.

Winter depression is a type of despondency that returns year after year during the winter period. Its symptoms appear in the autumn, and abate in the spring when the hours of daylight increase. Sufferers are characterized by their depressed mood, lack of concentration, sleep disturbances, and irritability. Fatigue, especially in the morning, is the major symptom. They sleep a great deal, especially during the day, but none the less lack energy and feel feeble and exhausted. The reason for this tiredness is that their sleep is disturbed thus not allowing the brain to recuperate.

Another symptom of winter depression is that appetite is enhanced. Many people feel a strong craving for carbohydrates, such as bread, pasta, and sweets, and weight gain is common among sufferers. Seasonal weight change is considered to be a greater problem amongst women than men.

Melatonin

The regulation of the sleep-wakefulness cycle is governed by the alternation between light and darkness and the secretion of a hormone called melatonin. Light curbs the production of melatonin and this helps to regulate our body clock. There is a natural connection between the hormone melatonin and another hormone known as cortisol, produced in a gland just above the kidney. Production of cortisol also shows a typical daily rhythm. Both these hormones influence mood regulation. In the depressed person a typical daily rhythm in the secretion of both melatonin and cortisol is disturbed.

Treating winter depression with light

Light therapy or 'bright-light therapy' (BLT) helps to reset the biological clock, by reducing melatonin secretion in the brain. This therapy has proved highly effective in winter depression; as many as 80% of sufferers become entirely free from symptoms.

The treatment is adapted to the individual patient's daily rhythm and may be given in the morning or evening, depending on whether the person concerned is a 'night owl' or an 'early bird'. The effects are usually noticeable after only a few treatment sessions. Light therapy is described in more detail in Chapter 18.

📄 Maria, aged 32: seasonal depression

Maria, who is 32 years old, works as a pharmaceutical representative in a major international company. She is an energetic person and gets a lot done at work. She is also active in her spare time, going to the gym several times a week. She seems to find time for everything—friends, husband, outdoor recreation, sport, and work. She is a cheerful, light-hearted person.

Over the past 2 years, however, she has begun to suffer from fatigue during the winter months. Every morning has become an ordeal. Her energy evaporates as soon as the November darkness settles. After struggling through a whole week's work, she is utterly exhausted and would prefer to sleep all weekend—like an urge to hibernate. Seeing friends does not tempt her and she does not feel well enough to go to the gym. She consumes large quantities of chocolate, which otherwise never appeals to her. She becomes fat and bloated during the dark winter months.

Maria does all she can to keep going so as not to lose out to competitors in her demanding job. She struggles on despite her evident tiredness and lack of commitment. Suddenly, one beautiful spring day, Maria feels a renewed urge to see her friends. She accompanies her husband and a few friends to the country and feels her joy and energy returning.

Maria's husband Peter talks to his mother-in-law about Maria's change of mood. Maria's mother is retired and spends half the year in Spain. When Peter talks about Maria's condition, her mother gives a smile of recognition: 'I've been like that for many years,' she says. 'That's why I used to take holidays in November, not in the summer like everyone else. I was able to travel to sunnier parts of the world and avoid feeling that terrible tiredness. Perhaps you two should consider taking a long sunny holiday next winter.'

4

Depression in childhood and adolescence

> ## ➔ Key points
>
> - It can be difficult for a parent to distinguish between ordinary signs of puberty or natural despondency and a depressive illness.
>
> - Depression manifests itself differently during adolescence: girls withdraw, boys become disruptive.
>
> - Common signs of depression in a child or adolescent are:
>
>   - Irritability and despondency
>
>   - Loss of joy, pleasure, and initiative
>
>   - Appetite/sleep disturbance
>
>   - Tiredness and lack of energy
>
>   - Changes in motor activity
>
>   - Low self-esteem and a sense of guilt
>
>   - Concentration difficulties
>
>   - Physical pains: stomach ache, frequent headaches etc.
>
>   - Anxiety
>
>   - Disruptive behaviour (in boys)
>
>   - Suicidality.

Children and adolescents can develop depression but often do not receive the care they need. This may be connected with the profound sense of guilt that sad children arouse in adults—which makes us reluctant to see and understand their suffering. It may also be because we have difficulty in believing that children and adolescents can become severely despondent.

A moment of patience can save us from the greatest misfortune.
A moment of impatience can destroy our whole life.

Chinese proverb

Children and adolescents

It is unusual for young children to become depressed. An estimated 0.2–2% of children develop depression before puberty, and it is equally common among boys and girls. After puberty despondency is three to four times more common in girls, and an estimated 3–4% of teenagers suffer from depression. Very often, it is difficult for a parent to distinguish between ordinary signs of puberty or natural despondency and a depressive illness.

Depression manifests itself differently in boys and girls. Depressed girls withdraw, are silent, or seem shy, and this may perhaps explain why adults often overlook their symptoms. In boys, depression may very often be the hidden, underlying cause of their disruptive behaviour. Depressed boys achieve less than others and can be rowdy, abuse alcohol, and offend people.

Common symptoms of depression in children and adolescents

Irritability and despondency

One common symptom of depression in the young is irritability, which may alternate with despondency. Despondency may be the only symptom the depressed child shows and it may continue for weeks, with fairly little variation from one day to the next. The depressed child may be less despondent in the evening. It is not unusual for depressed children to cry every day. Boys' rowdy behaviour may mask their depression.

Loss of joy, pleasure, and initiative

Depressed children lose their capacity to enjoy their usual activities. If the depression becomes more severe, young individuals may isolate themselves entirely from their peers and from the family. It is not unusual for severely despondent children and adolescents to have very poor contact with their friends as they cannot face being with others.

Appetite disturbances

Some depressed children console themselves by eating and put on weight, without enjoying what they eat, while other children lose their appetites, pick at their food, and eat too little. Among younger children, the normal weight gain fails to take place. Young people with anorexia (self-starvation) very often develop a depressive illness.

Sleep disturbances

Children and adolescents who are not depressed can compensate for their sleep deficiency and tiredness with a good night's sleep the following night. This does not apply to depressed children and adolescents, whose sleep disturbances are persistent, and who are tired and lethargic and do not feel rested, despite the many hours they spend in bed.

Tiredness and lack of energy

Depressed children and adolescents experience fatigue, and are worried and anxious about not having the strength to engage in activities that otherwise cause no problems for them.

Change in motor activity

Some depressed children and adolescents may become slow and sluggish. But this is far from the inhibited motor activity that may be seen in depressed adults. Agitation and excitement may characterize young depressed children.

Low self-esteem and sense of guilt

Low self-esteem is a common symptom of depression in the young. Depressed girls do not like either their appearance or their personality. Sometimes they may even hate themselves. Depressed adolescents may also suffer from marked feelings of guilt. They may, for example, believe that they are the cause of their parents' divorce or some other discord in the family. Young people who are normally conscientious and perfectionist may incur a strong sense of guilt when they are severely despondent, because of all the duties they cannot manage to perform.

Concentration difficulties

Depressed children and adolescents often have attention disorders and difficulties in concentrating. They find it hard to listen and sit still, are easily distracted, and do not complete tasks they have begun. As a rule, depressed children perform relatively poorly at school, do not bond with their classmates, and appear aimless. It is estimated that half of truancy can be attributed to depression.

Pain

Frequent headaches, stomach ache, and shooting pains in the legs or chest, may be a sign of depression in the young.

Anxiety

Depression in the young may often be accompanied by severe anxiety. Some despondent adolescents try to stop their anguish and treat their own depression with alcohol. In the short term, alcohol can reduce anxiety and alleviate symptoms of depression. However, in the long term the depression is not cured and the anxiety fails to disappear; instead, all the negative social and psychological consequences of alcohol abuse make their appearance.

Suicidal thoughts and attempted suicide

Suicidal thoughts are very common among children and adolescents who are depressed, although suicide attempts are much less common. There is a discrepancy between the way in which depressed children experience and describe their situation and their parents' perceptions. Parents often describe their depressed children as disobedient, restless, irritable, tearful, disruptive, and quarrelsome. Depressed children and adolescents describe themselves as sad, unhappy, and pessimistic. They are filled with anguish and have negative perceptions of their body.

Causes of depression in children and adolescents

Natural despondency in children may occur as part of normal development when, for example, they start school or enter their teens. Loss is, in normal cases, part of human development. Depression develops only in certain individuals and very seldom has a single cause: it is a multifactorial illness.

If either of a child's parents is or has been depressed, the risk of the child also developing a depression increases almost fourfold. If both the parents have depression, the risk rises tenfold. Besides biological inheritance, the mother's or father's depression is perceived by the child not only as a chronic stressor but also as a kind of 'life model' for how to react to life's tribulations.

Poor relationships with parents may also contribute to a sense of being under chronic stress. In families where the parents are depressed, suffer from another mental illness, or are substance abusers, their responsiveness to the children's needs is often poor. The child may then develop a feeling of hopelessness. Learned helplessness in the child may also be due to the parents' constant dissatisfaction with the child, regardless of what they do, how they behave or what they achieve. This learned feeling of helplessness, which impairs a person's capacity for action, accompanies the child into adult life.

However, there are exceptions to every rule. Many children who grow up with depressed parents do not themselves become depressed. They may, instead, develop a particular sensitivity to the needs of others. As they learnt to look after both themselves and the depressed parent at an early stage, they may become unusually strong and stable adults. Such people often seek occupations connected with health and social care, and frequently prove empathetic and skilful in their work.

Active children manage to find good models outside the family and, accordingly, good coping strategies even if they grow up in emotional deprivation. Many child-abuse 'survivors' cope well with the trauma and become successful in both their social and their professional lives. However, among child abuse survivors, there may be deep wounds that, in stressful situations, may re-open. It is not unusual for a person who has long resisted stress and difficulties, to succumb finally to depression. This depression may be played down by both the sufferer and others, as everyone has been accustomed to the person coping well in spite of difficulties.

The most common precipitating causes of depression and natural despondency in children and adolescents include:

- ◆ **Loss**: Of a parent or person whom the young individual feels close to and loves. Loss of a boyfriend or girlfriend, especially if there was a sexual relationship, can spark off severe despondency.

- ◆ **Disappointments**: Not being admitted to a study course, or failing an examination or competition to which they have devoted a great deal of effort. Other causes may be getting poorer than expected grades, or feeling let down by people who are dear to them.

- ◆ **Traumatic life events**: Such as mental or physical abuse, sexual exploitation, and bullying. The parents' substance abuse or lasting mental or physical illness, relationship problems in the family and family financial problems are examples of other negative life events.

◆ **Infant depression**: Illness, physical disability, chronic illness, or a severe infection can cause depression in some children and adolescents. Clinical observations of infants also show that, even in the first year of life, they can develop what is clearly depression after being separated from their mothers. Depression is manifested in the form of passivity, inactivity, sorrow, and stereotyped movements, i.e. rocking back and forth with an empty look in their eyes. On the basis of these observations, small children are not nowadays admitted to hospital alone, without the company of one or both parents. The purpose of this is to prevent depression, which impedes the healing process.

Sound self-esteem: a protective factor

Good self-esteem in children is known to be a factor protecting them against depression. Self-esteem develops from children's and parents' mutual communication. If the parent–child relationship works well, the child feels seen and appreciated. Through loving but firm limits with clearly expressed values and norms, parents lay the foundations of well-being in children and help them to develop harmoniously with a strong self-esteem.

Supportive parents can encourage reserved and withdrawn children to cautiously seek contact and make friends, to offset their tendencies towards isolation. They can sensitively stimulate and encourage the child. If parents disregard their children's withdrawn disposition, their social development and contact with friends may suffer.

Advice to parents and other adults

Parents have their own life histories, problems, and limitations, which influence their relations with their children and how they cope with looking after a depressed child. Living with a depressed child may be difficult. Life changes completely, and family life becomes chaotic.

As a parent, one may sometimes feel inadequate. However, talking to other adults about the situation and sense of inadequacy affords relief. If a parent feels unable to give sufficient support to a child, other adults may step in instead. The essentials are to care for the child, seek support from other adults, and venture to apply for professional help.

Negative stress and trauma support

When dealing with depressed children and adolescents, parents and teachers must ensure that the impact of negative life events is alleviated and worked through. They must also ensure that the stress to which children are exposed, or feel that they are exposed, is eliminated. It is not the intensity and degree of a traumatic life event that is most important, but the child's way of experiencing such an event. Some children feel that very small changes in their life are severe tribulations, while others have a much greater stress tolerance.

Children and adolescents have a great capacity to recover from and repair the damage of traumatic events they have experienced. They can recover from the most atrocious traumas, such as incest or torture, if they receive help in working through these events. A recuperative process should preferably start immediately after the trauma and continue as the child grows up, but help in later life may also yield positive results.

Teach children to take their feelings seriously

Children who lack a broad range of action alternatives and have poor strategies for coping with difficulties often feel chronic stress and may develop depression. It is therefore important to teach children to acknowledge their problems and talk to others.

Children should also be encouraged to confide in other adults outside the family circle: perhaps a teacher or recreation leader whom they trust. Children's chances of coping with depression are greater when they talk about their problems than when they bottle up their emotions.

Make time to spend with the children

In talking to a depressed child or young person, one should not allow oneself to be distracted by anything else. It is important for the young person to feel that they are the sole object of attention. Children should not be reproached for their depression, nor told to pull themselves together or cheer up. By pushing and exerting pressure on children, one imposes strain on them. It is wrong to believe that children can be made to change in the course of a depression by means of reprimands.

Provide the right amount of stimulation

'Letting the child or young person be' during a depression is not the right way to help. Depressed adolescents need encouragement and support to be active and seek their friends' company, and not merely sink down apathetically in front of the television. Withdrawn children with a depressive disposition can learn that they do not need many friends; one friend can be enough.

One should not hesitate to provide practical assistance with schoolwork, cooking, or whatever activity the child enjoyed before becoming despondent.

A depressed child who has lost all pleasure and interest in ordinary activities needs stimulation. Do not allow the child to become isolated. It is difficult to know how much to leave the depressed young individual in peace, and how much to stimulate and exert pressure. If it is difficult to engage the child in a joint activity, it may be enough for someone to be in the same room, sitting together on the sofa. Physical proximity can give depressed children security and the strength to establish a more active rapport, in due course, with their parents or others.

Show that you are fond of the child

Children must feel that their parents are fond of them. This must be shown not only by words, but also by physical contact, i.e. hugs and kisses. It is not wrong to impose reasonable demands on depressed young people if they simultaneously feel loved. Praise and encouragement when children have done something good are just as important as loving, constructive criticism when they have done something wrong. The essential thing is for children and adolescents to feel that their parents accept and like them regardless of how they themselves feel and what they do.

Give the same amount of attention to each child

Sometimes it is difficult to give equal attention to all the children within a family. Parents are often aware of this and try to divide their time, energy, and attention equally. Nevertheless, children who are ill or depressed often monopolize the family's attention. All concentration is focused on the despondent individual. It is therefore important for the depressed child's siblings to receive attention as well, as they also run the risk of developing depression.

Treatment of depression in the young

Parents should never hesitate to seek professional help. It is difficult to break the vicious circle that exists in families with depressed children, which contributes to the uncertainty and irresolution.

Treatment of children and adolescents who are depressed should always be supervised by a specialist in child and adolescent psychiatry. Most children and adolescents regain their health by means of psychotherapy alone. Cognitive psychotherapy and interpersonal psychotherapy—combined with family therapy—are the forms of treatment normally used for children and adolescents. It is important for children to be treated with their families to permit a change in the family dynamics, and to teach the parents how to cope with family life with a depressed child.

Treatment with antidepressants is given to children and adolescents only in cases of severe depression, and then always in combination with psychotherapy. The crucial point to remember is that children and adolescents, as well as adults, receiving treatment with antidepressants should be cautiously monitored for side-effects, signs of anxiety, and suicidal thoughts. The possible risk of elevated suicidality must always be weighed against expected improvement during the treatment.

During treatment, depressed adolescents often rapidly gain an insight into how their irritability and despondency affects their parents and others. However, it may take a long time for children to learn to change their behaviour. Here, patience is called for from parents, teachers, and schoolmates. Cooperation with the school is important, as is informing teachers about the child's depression and treatment arrangements.

Mathew, aged 16: depression

Mathew has always been retiring, but in senior school (age 13–15) he began to be perceived as an 'odd boy'. His former friends spent all their spare time on sport or outdoor recreation. Mathew did not enjoy such activities, and became increasingly lonely. At home, he was silent and tended to shut himself into his room and read. He often quarrelled with his father. The parents fought a great deal between themselves, and Mathew heard them talk about divorce. At weekends, the quarrels became more heated—partly because they drank too much alcohol.

During his first term at upper secondary school, Mathew's state of health deteriorated steadily. He was tired, and felt angry with everything and everyone. He belittled himself, regarding himself as 'a nobody'. Everything felt pointless. The need to withdraw grew increasingly strong, and he no longer had any friends. Once, when Mathew was to read aloud in a French lesson, he was unable to get a word out and, stammering, rushed out of the classroom. His studies went from bad to worse. Mathew had every possible excuse for not going to school—headache, stomach ache, 'crazy' teachers, etc. When these did not help, he began playing truant and drifted around aimlessly in the streets.

The teachers contacted Mathew's parents, who raised the problem with him. This discussion resulted in a vehement quarrel, with shouting, crying, and Mathew threatening to take his own life. He then ran out, slamming the front door after him. After a few hours the father found

Mathew, whimpering inconsolably on a park bench with a bottle of spirits beside him. 'If this happens again, you may just as well move away from home!' shouted his father angrily. Mathew went home with his father, but family relations were extremely strained. His father was hardly ever at home, his mother had given up her attempts to get close to Mathew, and his sister did not seem to care about him.

One day the school welfare officer telephoned Mathew and suggested a meeting. Mathew protested and wondered what good it would do, but the counsellor insisted. Reluctantly, Mathew promised to meet her. The meeting was a turning point for him. Despite his resistance, he realized that the welfare officer was a person who wanted to try and help him. Mathew has now been attending psychotherapy for 1 year. He has moved away from home and left school. He still cannot cope with too many demands. He lives with a distant relative, and helps out in a car-repair shop in the daytime. His future plans are still diffuse. But he feels better and less heavy-hearted. Sometimes he tells his therapist that his supreme wish—if only he could concentrate and bring himself to resume his studies—is to work with children in the future.

5

Women, men, and depression

 Key points

◆ Male depression is often masked by alcohol consumption, irritability, aggression, and violence.

◆ Depressed men do not usually talk about anguish, sadness, or despondency. They refer to work problems and difficulties in concentration.

◆ Women find it easier to describe their own moods, and therefore have a greater capacity to seek help—this also helps professionals to diagnose depression and help women.

◆ Psychosomatic ailments and pain of various types can be symptoms of depression in women.

◆ If a woman is already depressed, she usually feels worse during the premenstrual period.

◆ Most women have a sense of emotional well-being when they are pregnant; however, after childbirth, some succumb to a natural feeling of despondency known as 'maternity blues'.

Women run a higher risk of becoming depressed than men. There are various explanations for this difference. One reason why depression is more easily diagnosed in women is that women express mental symptoms verbally, more often than men.

Symptoms of depression in men and women

There is a difference between how depression is expressed in men and women. Male depression is masked by alcohol consumption, increased aggression, and violence. Men who suffer from depression develop symptoms that are fewer than those of women. Depressed men frequently refer to their poor concentration and to deterioration in occupational situations. A depressed man does not usually talk about anguish, sadness, or despondency.

Women find it easier to describe their own moods, and therefore have a greater capacity to seek help, making it easier for doctors to make diagnoses. Psychosomatic ailments and pain of various types are often symptoms of female depression. Anguish, panic attacks, and signs of phobia also occur more often in women than in men. Moreover, the 'atypical depressions'—characterized by an increased sleep requirement and an enhanced appetite, with visible weight gain—are more common in women.

Caroline, aged 45: a woman heading for depression

Caroline is an economics graduate, married to an engineer. The couple have an adolescent daughter called Sophie, and also a 20-year-old daughter, Anne, who has recently moved away from home. Caroline has several siblings, and her aged parents live fairly close by. Caroline has always been cheerful, helpful, and nurturing. She always does her best to help her brothers and sisters when they are in need, and visits her own and her husband's parents almost every weekend. As a child, too, she was competent and energetic, helpful and positive. She particularly helped her mother, who often had problems because of the father's alcoholism. Caroline's friends liked her and sought her company. However, Caroline often felt sad when she was alone in the evenings.

Caroline's father developed Alzheimer's disease, and a few years ago her mother decided to look after him at home. After work, Caroline started going to visit her parents daily to help her mother. Her siblings did not become involved in caring for their father as Caroline had voluntarily assumed this responsibility.

Her father's illness went on for several years, and Caroline neglected both her own home and her daughter. One day, Caroline received a call from the emergency social-welfare authorities. Sophie had been found on a park bench under the influence of marijuana and alcohol. Caroline was utterly dismayed. She became insomniac and fell prey to an almost bottomless sense of hopelessness. Only then did her husband and siblings realize that they must help to relieve the burden on Caroline. The family convened for a crisis meeting and drew up a schedule for care of the father and mother. Caroline was freed from duties regarding her parents. However, she continued to feel poorly, was reluctant to meet any friends, became very introspective, and stopped eating.

Within a couple of weeks, she had developed profound melancholia. She could not bring herself to go to family therapy with her drug-addicted daughter. The district physician prescribed antidepressants, and her husband had to take leave from work. He supported Caroline, and their daughter was temporarily placed with relatives in the country. After 2 months Caroline started feeling better, but she had difficulty in finding her old happy self. Sophie had to stay with the relatives in the countryside for another term. During the summer the family took a long holiday, and at the end of the summer they embarked on family therapy.

Depressions specific to women

Premenstrual complaints and tension

In the days preceding menstruation, many women feel despondent. Most women—up to 75%—experience tiredness and irritability, with mild mental and physical symptoms. The mental symptoms include anxiety, dejected mood, increased susceptibility to exhaustion, and concentration difficulties. The physical symptoms include feeling bloated, with tightness in the breasts and extremities. Headache, frequent urination, and an increased tendency to sweat are common.

Premenstrual syndrome

Premenstrual syndrome starts in the week before menstruation and ceases roughly 24 hours after menstruation starts. The symptoms usually disappear a week after menstruation. If a woman is already depressed, she usually feels worse during the premenstrual period. Suicide attempts may occur during this period. This applies particularly to depressed women who are substance abusers.

Premenstrual dysphoric disorder

During the week before menstruation, 2.5–5% of women feel so ill that they fulfil the criteria required for premenstrual dysphoric disorder to be diagnosed.

The symptoms, which may recur regularly during most menstrual cycles, are severe and characterized by:

◆ marked despondency and anxiety

◆ sharply reduced interest in ordinary activities

◆ increased susceptibility to exhaustion

◆ emotional liability with lack of self-control

◆ severe irritability

◆ rage (in the most extreme cases).

Broken marriages or ruined relationships with other family members, friends, and co-workers are not uncommon for women with premenstrual dysphoric disorder. It commonly starts at the age of 30–45, and ends with the menopause. Very often, the symptoms worsen after childbirth.

Treatment of premenstrual syndrome and premenstrual dysphoric disorder

Mild premenstrual complaints may be relieved by physical exercise, which reduces the accumulation of fluid in the body and also helps to reduce tiredness. It is crucial to take the symptoms seriously—massage and rest may help to relieve symptoms. The most severe form of premenstrual trouble, premenstrual dysphoric disorder, is reminiscent of the disturbances suffered by a depressed person, and can be treated with antidepressants.

Contraceptive pills and depression

In sufferers from severe premenstrual syndrome and premenstrual dysphoric disorder in particular, depression may be precipitated by the Pill. The newer contraceptives in use today contain very small quantities of hormones. But these pills, too, may have depression-inducing effects in women who suffer from severe premenstrual syndrome or premenstrual dysphoric disorder, or who have previously been deeply despondent.

The menopause and depression

In 95% of women, the menopause starts between the ages of 42 and 58. During the menopause, some women have physical symptoms such as sweating, hot flushes, and dry genital membranes. They are also troubled by tiredness, despondency, irritability, and reduced sexual desire (libido). Roughly 25%

of women are free from symptoms or have very mild ailments during the menopause. In some women, on the other hand, the symptoms may persist for up to 15 years after the menopause begins.

Oestrogen and well-being

Oestrogen is known to have mood-elevating effects. Ordinary oestrogen-replacement therapy for menopause problems has marked positive effects on anxiety, despondency, sleep, energy, and sexual relations.

Risks of oestrogen treatment

There are risks associated with treating women with oestrogen (hormone replacement therapy (HRT)). They may, for example, develop breast cancer or blood clots. There is also some risk of developing cancer in the lining of the uterus. It is essential for women receiving oestrogen treatment to undergo regular medical checks. Women with cancer, pronounced obesity, heart failure, and severe varicose veins, and those of advanced age, should not be treated with oestrogen.

At present, oestrogen treatment may be recommended for women who, during the menopause, are troubled by hot flushes, sweating, palpitations, and also dry and fragile membranes in the urogenital system, and to prevent brittleness of the bones (osteoporosis). Women who are taking oestrogen are encouraged to undergo regular medical check-ups, to exercise regularly, and to adopt a varied and nutritious diet. It is also important to stop smoking.

Pregnancy, childbirth, and depression

Most women have a strong sense of emotional well-being when they are pregnant. After childbirth, however, many succumb to a natural feeling of despondency or a short-lived depressive reaction known as 'maternity blues'. A more severe form of depression after childbirth, known as postpartum depression (PPD), occurs in about 10–15% of women who have recently given birth. Another serious condition that may arise after the birth is postpartum psychosis that arises in about 0.1% of women.

Maternity blues

There are both psychological and biological reasons why pregnant women feel good. Oestrogen and progesterone levels, which are very high during pregnancy, contribute to pregnant women's mental well-being. After childbirth, the oestrogen and the progesterone fall to their normal pre-pregnancy levels. This sudden fall in the two hormones may cause emotional instability in the new mother, and a brief depressive reaction. A temporary, short-lived down-turn in mood occurs in many women who have recently given birth. This is entirely normal and reaches its peak 5 days after the birth and ceases after a week to 10 days; unlike PPD.

An attack of 'maternity blues' is characterized by slight despondency and emotional instability. The new mother cries easily, may be extremely sensitive and tired, may have difficulty in falling asleep and in concentrating. Irritability is another striking symptom. Alternatively, some women enter an euphoric state and become elated after childbirth.

Postpartum depression (PPD)

PPD (also known as postnatal depression), arises in considerably fewer women, within 4 weeks after childbirth. Sleep disturbances, markedly low self-confidence, irritability, and restlessness are conspicuous symptoms. A depressed new mother sleeps poorly and is generally fragile. She may cry one moment and laugh the next. Sometimes, she may fear harming the baby and herself and may not want to take care of the baby. Women who have had a previous depressive illness are at risk of developing PPD and should therefore receive medical and psychological support during pregnancy.

Postpartum paternal depression

PPD may develop not only in mothers, but in fathers too. Paternal depression can adversely affect a child's behavioural and emotional development and there is an elevated risk of depression and suicide behaviours in the offspring of parents with depression.

Postpartum psychosis

Postpartum psychosis is experienced by 1 in 1000 women after childbirth. The onset is within 2 weeks to 1 month after the birth, often with mania or rapidly alternating depressive and manic phases. Women who have a manic-depressive illness may suffer a relapse after childbirth. A depression with psychotic confusion occurs more often in women over the age of 30 giving birth for the first time. Hallucinations and delusions are common. The latter often focus on the baby and the mother's fear of hurting it. Postpartum psychosis requires hospital treatment.

📄 Margaret, aged 35: postpartum psychosis

Margaret and Philip lived in a London suburb. Philip had his own small firm and worked as an electrician, while Margaret was employed as a pre-school teacher. They both liked children and had always wanted to have their own. Unfortunately, Margaret had suffered two consecutive miscarriages and, after several years of marriage, they had almost given up hope. One summer while Margaret was away visiting her mother, Philip was tempted into having an affair with a neighbour's wife, and at the same time it emerged that Margaret was pregnant. After painful scenes, they both reached the conclusion that they wanted to keep the baby and live together. After all, they were very fond of each other and got on well together.

The pregnancy proceeded according to plan, but suddenly, a week after the birth, Margaret broke out in vehement accusations against Philip. She would pour out the most extreme accusations, only to apologise a few hours later. This went on: one moment, as Margaret saw it, their relationship was worthless and they might as well break up, and the next she had great plans for their joint future.

Her outbursts got worse and worse. Finally, both Philip and Margaret realized that she had to seek help. Margaret was put in touch with a psychologist in an outpatient department, with whom she had a few sessions on her own. The psychologist talked to Philip only fleetingly on a single occasion. The sessions made Margaret feel better, but just a few weeks later the situation deteriorated once more. Margaret suffered from severe attacks of anguish. She got worked up, and ran round turning up the volume of the television and stereo, and so forth. Every sensation—everything she saw, heard, and tasted—felt heightened. Her thoughts became oppressive, she had difficulty in concentrating on anything, and she was constantly afraid of hurting the baby and Philip.

The doctors decided that she should be committed to a psychiatric ward. However, Philip was not properly informed about Margaret's illness and how she was to be treated. When Margaret came home from hospital she was, at first, subdued; but after a month or so her vehement accusations against Philip about his affair with the neighbour's wife began once again, alternating with assurances that she loved him. It turned out later that Margaret had been given medication at the hospital, but had stopped taking it as soon as she got home. As Philip had not been informed about her medication, he did not know what was wrong. The emotional roller-coaster began again. Times when everything was wonderful and could not have been better were followed by periods of the deepest despair and depression. The couple sought help once more.

Philip and Margaret attended family therapy together and, at the same time, Margaret was treated with medication and regained her health. They devote a great deal of time to each other and their child. Family life is important to them both.

Treatment of depression in pregnant women and new mothers

It is vital for a pregnant woman's depression to be treated, as several studies have shown that there are marked adverse psychological repercussions on the child if the mother is depressed. Children of depressed mothers have more difficulty in establishing relationships with their classmates and members of the opposite sex and perform less well at school. They also have an elevated risk of succumbing to depression.

Antidepressants

The choice of treatment is based on an assessment of the mother's mental state and the risks to the mother and fetus entailed by the absence of treatment. Antidepressants are not usually harmful to the mother, but some are suspected of possible effects on the fetus or of causing withdrawal and toxic symptoms in the baby during delivery. The established practice is to avoid antidepressants as far as possible during pregnancy and use other biological forms of treatment in severe depressions combined with psychosocial and psychological interventions.

6

The elderly and depression

➜ Key points

◆ Among the elderly (those aged 70 and over) depressions are fairly common but often undiagnosed; so many cases of depression go untreated.

◆ People who have not previously been depressed may become severely despondent when they are old as their life situation alters, often due to sudden solitude.

◆ Some medicines prescribed for physical ailments may trigger despondency and depression.

◆ Some typical symptoms of depression in the elderly are: strong tiredness, physical ailments, striking weight loss, weariness, anxiety, anguish, and insomnia.

◆ The risk of suicide is high in the elderly, especially among those who live alone.

◆ Relatives, care services, and friends all play a key role in supporting elderly people.

◆ Good medical care, company, a nutritious diet, and stimulating activities are vital for a good quality of life in old age.

How we perceive our own age varies between individuals, depending partly on our hereditary, biological characteristics, and partly on our psychosocial situation and psychological perceptions. In old age one may get depressed, although one has never been before.

Depression in the elderly

With advancing age, most people find new roles and new ways of life. Many are happy about finding more time to devote to activities they neglected during their working lives. But for some, ageing is a lonely, monotonous wait for nothing.

Among the elderly (defined as those aged 70 and over), depressions are fairly common but often undiagnosed, thus many cases of depression go untreated. People who live alone or in nursing homes, retirement homes, or geriatric wards manifest signs of depression on a much larger scale. In many cases, these states of depression are due not solely to biological ageing, but also to psychological causes. These may include lack of stimulation, interest, and attention.

Changes in brain function

Depression is often a consequence of age-related changes in the central nervous system and reduced activity in brain systems. These systems play a crucial part in regulating our emotional life and moods. One typical example of an illness that affects the central nervous system and is often accompanied by depression is Parkinson's disease. Alzheimer's disease sufferers also show a high prevalence of major depression.

Depression and senile dementia

Depression may sometimes occur in people who have dementia. Depressed people with symptoms of dementia may be touchy, easily moved to tears, and also tormented by nocturnal anguish. Sometimes sedatives are of no help: instead, they increase anxiety.

In dementia where depression is simultaneously present, the elderly person shows marked anxiety and certain personality changes. The patient may feel jealous and show paranoid symptoms that may, for example, take the form of suspicions that someone wants to get into their home and steal things. Depression in people suffering from dementia usually improves on treatment with antidepressants or electroconvulsive treatment (ECT).

Psychosocial factors

People who have not previously been depressed may become severely despondent when they are old. Many depressions in the elderly are due to the totally transformed life situation they encounter, often due to sudden solitude. They may feel lonely even if they are being cared for. The days are long. Their eating may worsen without anyone noticing, the metabolism decreases, and the organs of the body function more slowly. The person slowly slips into a state of dejection, and in due course a protracted depression.

Many elderly people are subjected to stress from the death of a family member. Dependence on other people (often strangers), lack of contact with close relatives, and limited financial resources are other examples of stressors. People who have concentrated solely on their jobs and not developed any other activities or interests may succumb to dejection on retirement. People with obsessive dependence on routine may become depressed when they stop working, until they have had time to develop new routines.

Physical illnesses and medications

Physical illnesses with their associated pain, such as reduced mobility, impaired vision and hearing, and poor sleep may result in the emergence of depression. Dietary deficiencies of such substances as fatty acids, vitamin B_{12}, and folic acid, which are essential for adequate brain function, may also cause depression.

One may become depressed from certain medicines that are used or suddenly withdrawn when treating physical illnesses. Certain combinations of medicines may trigger despondency and depression. As treatment with several different drugs is extremely common among the elderly, it is important for the person themselves, or their relatives, to tell the doctor which medicines have been prescribed previously. The doctor can then eliminate drugs that may possibly cause a depression, or replace them with an alternative drug.

It is common for elderly people to not always have their cupboards in order, and sometimes to accidentally take medicines that they no longer need. It is also a good idea for people themselves, or their relatives, to clear out the medicine cupboard at regular intervals.

Symptoms of depression in the elderly

Symptoms of depression in the elderly are often overshadowed by physical ailments such as: strong tiredness, headache, aches in muscles, joints, spine, stomach, bowel, heart problems such as palpitations, dizziness, and shortness of breath—and this may make it difficult for a doctor to make the right diagnosis.

Striking weight loss is a typical symptom of depression in elderly people. The course of the illness is often subtle, and many people therefore believe that the symptoms of depression are a manifestation of ageing instead.

Hypochondria is an exaggerated and unjustified worry, anxiety, and even severe anguish concerning physical health and is very common among the elderly. Other signs of depression in the elderly are a marked anxiety about financial issues, even if finances are sound.

The causes of insomnia, which is a common symptom of depression at any age, often has connections with unjustified and exaggerated daily worries. Elderly people need less sleep in the first place, and they also wake up frequently at night owing to the recurrent need to urinate, which obviously disturbs sleep. In addition, elderly people often sleep in the daytime, which reduces their need for nocturnal sleep.

A typical course of depression in the elderly is for the person to feel well for a few days, or even a few weeks, and thereafter lapse into a new period of depression. These mood 'dips' are particularly hard to bear. Moreover, during the period when they feel well, people believe that their depressive symptoms will not recur and therefore postpone consulting a doctor.

Treatment of depression in the elderly

The elderly usually respond well to antidepressant treatment but, as a rule, need long-term medication. This is because the symptoms are often more chronic. Elderly individuals are more sensitive to medicines and suffer from more side effects than younger people. Treatment should therefore always start with a low dose of antidepressants that can be increased.

Overall, the elderly need continuous and loving care, which cannot be replaced solely by medicines or other forms of therapy. Support and continuity of care are vital for all people, but particularly important for elderly people, who are often on their own, and heavily dependent on others.

Relatives' roles

As a relative one can provide support, care, and stimulation. In consultation with the home-help service, or day health-care facilities, relatives can help the depressed person to find suitable forms of treatment and rehabilitation. A doctor should be contacted as soon as the person begins to become dejected, sleeps or eats poorly, or generally seems different.

If a doctor diagnoses a patient as depressed, one should always ask about treatment and what is expected of family members. The most important task is to encourage the depressed person to complete a course of treatment, and not to give up if the effects are not immediately noticeable. It usually takes time before the depressive symptoms and signs of anxiety subside, sometimes several months. In psychological forms of treatment, it takes longer for symptoms to be decreased.

Day centres, walks, physiotherapy, massage, hot baths, excursions, or such pursuits that the elderly person enjoys have a stimulating and cheering effect. Once or twice a week is usually enough; otherwise it may be an effort for the elderly person, who has limited physical endurance and mental capacity to respond to external stimulation.

One should ensure that the elderly person eats properly prepared and nutritious meals containing fibre-rich and high-protein foods, vitamins, and minerals. A good diet prevents anaemia and provides important amino acids. More advice to relatives is given in Chapter 20.

Suicide risk in the elderly

Anxiety is a common manifestation of depression in the elderly. Antidepressant treatment may initially increase anxiety. During this initial period when anxiety is increasing, the risk of suicidal acts is great. Particular attention and surveillance on the part of relatives and care staff is therefore required. Anxiety may be relieved by sedatives during this initial period. The risk of suicide is high in the elderly, especially those who live alone and are socially isolated. If an elderly person has been depressed for a long time, there is a major risk of suicide attempts in the event of sudden psychological and social trauma or a changed life situation.

7

Physical illness, pain, symptoms, and depression

 Key points

- Physical illnesses that may lead to severe despondency include; cancer, rheumatism, chronic asthma, chronic respiratory infections, cardiac infarction, and anaemia.

- Physical illnesses may change people's lives and restrict both their professional and social activities which may induce depression.

- Certain illnesses, such as epilepsy, stroke, Parkinson's disease, and multiple sclerosis (MS), attack and damage parts of the brain with the consequence that sufferers may become depressed.

- Depression may sometimes be expressed through pain or physical symptoms without any underlying physical illness or organ damage.

- As many medicines can trigger depression, it is important for people to inform their doctors about existing medication when seeking help.

Physical diseases can impact on the functioning of the nervous system which can cause depression. There are also illnesses that indirectly, owing to their long duration or the resulting pain, bring about a marked change in a sufferer's quality of life leading to despondency and depression. Depression may also be concealed behind pain and physical symptoms, without any underlying illness.

Physical illness and depression

Many physical illnesses change people's lives and restrict both their professional and social activities. The changes involved are often so sweeping that the illness may induce either single depressive symptoms or full-blown depression.

Physical illnesses that may lead to severe despondency include cancer, rheumatism, chronic asthma, chronic respiratory infections, cardiac infarction, and anaemia. It is well known that patients that have undergone cardiac bypass surgery can develop depressive symptoms following the operation.

Depression due to pain

Acutely painful conditions very seldom result in despondency or depression. Chronic pain is defined as pain that has lasted for more than 6 months. In many cases, the chronic physical illness is accompanied by persistent pain impairing everyday life activities. The sufferer then runs a high risk of developing depression, and adequate treatment of chronic pain is therefore important.

Psychosomatic symptoms and depression

Depression may be masked with pain or physical symptoms, without any underlying illness or organ damage. The most common types of pain are located in the head, neck, back, joints, various muscles and, in women, the pelvic region. Others may complain of stomach ache, diarrhoea or constipation, nausea, itching, shooting pains in the heart region, palpitations, tiredness, weakness, dizziness, back or neck pain, numbness of the arms and legs, or a sensation of pressure in the head. In their pessimism, people may interpret these manifestations as indicating some serious or life-threatening physical illness.

Despite a thorough physical investigation, the doctor may not find any sign of physical illness. Sometimes, for people who mask their depression with pain or psychosomatic symptoms, it may take several years before a correct diagnosis is made. Instead of carrying out a psychological investigation, doctors prescribe various physical tests. Relatives, too, may concentrate on the depressed person's physical state. People with symptoms of this kind often have difficulty in expressing themselves and describing their life situation. For these people, it is easier to refer to pain or physical symptoms than to describe their emotions, anguish, and mental problems.

Psychosomatic ailments may be seen as a form of non-verbal language, signalling that something is wrong. Although, frequently, no immediate reason for the symptoms is apparent, a systematic review of a person's development and life situation may reveal hidden conflicts that may be suspected of causing depression. These symptoms may be a way of reacting to a life situation that people cannot cope with. The symptoms often improve when the depressed person is given a chance to express in words how they experience their own situation.

Often, it is people who pay relatively little attention to mental and emotional processes who express their psychological conflicts by physical symptoms. However, inability to get in touch with one's own experiences is not the only cause. Physical symptoms are not encumbered with prejudices to the same extent as psychiatric illnesses. Having a physical illness is, in many cultures, more acceptable than suffering from a mental one.

Depression concealed by other illnesses

Substance abuse, anguish, and compulsive syndromes may also mask depression. Depressions that arise in conjunction with these conditions usually improve considerably in response to either antidepressants or combinations of antidepressants and psychological forms of treatment.

Depression due to prescription medicines

Certain prescription medicines may contribute to despondency or the development of depression, or cause an existing depressive state to worsen. As many medicines can trigger depression, it is important for people to inform their doctors about their medication. A doctor who is fully informed can easily find out which medicine may have triggered the depression, and replace it. If one has a physical illness, it is also important to say if one has previously been depressed, so that the doctor can avoid prescribing drugs known for their capacity to induce depression.

Christine, aged 71: depression and physical illness

Christine was a heavy smoker of many years' standing. Throughout her working life, she had been a teacher. The work was stressful, and being able to smoke and relax very often afforded pleasurable relief. Her husband Peter, a headmaster, was also a heavy smoker.

After her retirement, Christine began to suffer from chest pain—initially just once a week or so, but eventually almost every day when she was out shopping, for example. Finally, she stopped going out when the weather was cold or windy, as the pain in her chest was so severe. She was also tired and short of breath, and her legs ached. Peter persuaded her to see the general practitioner, and after thorough investigations angina (severe chest pain) was diagnosed and medication was prescribed to relieve her symptoms.

One day, suddenly, Christine felt very tired and broke out in a cold sweat. There was no severe pain in her chest, but her appearance made it clear that something was wrong and she felt quite different from usual. She was 'ebbing away', and Peter immediately drove her to hospital. There, she was found to be having a heart attack. A contrast X-ray revealed severe constriction of the heart vessels (coronary vessels) and the doctor suggested surgery.

Despite anxiety, Christine decided to undergo surgery. The operation went well, and after only 10 days she was able to look after herself. The hospital social worker offered to arrange accommodation at a convalescent home, but Christine chose to go home.

Christine complied well with her physician's recommendations and took care to attend all the routine checks, take her medication, and follow the few instructions she was given concerning future activities. Her mood seemed, if anything, more cheerful than usual. However, about a month after her operation Christine suddenly began finding it difficult to get up in the morning, and complained that the operation scar was hurting. Low-spirited and discouraged, she slept poorly and fitfully, and was very often unable to fall asleep again after waking at about three or four in the morning. Her gloom deepened, and she lost the will to attend physiotherapy. She was unwilling even to see her general practitioner, whom she normally liked. Slowly the depression overwhelmed her and was increasingly obvious. Peter decided to wait and see how it developed. He did not want to worry Christine, and thought perhaps it was simply a delayed shock reaction to the major operation she had undergone. Nevertheless, when several weeks had passed and Christine was still hardly inclined to get out of bed, Peter contacted the district nurse.

The nurse visited them at home and talked to Christine. Christine was reluctant and felt tired, but finally loosened up and began to talk. She told the nurse that she had felt the same after giving birth to her first child, Elisabeth. Peter, too, remembered how depressed Christine had been after Elisabeth's birth and how she had improved greatly after electroconvulsive treatment. The district nurse said it was not unusual for people—and especially women who had previously suffered from depression at one time or other—to become depressed after a bypass operation.

Christine was given antidepressant medication. The doctor chose an antidepressant that did not interact with other medicines that Christine was taking. The doctor also changed Christine's medication to lower blood pressure, as the drugs she had previously been taking were known for their capacity to induce depression. Not until a year later did Christine feel more or less her old self again, and by the time another year had passed, she had entirely recovered from her depression and was able to enjoy her liberation from chest pain thanks to the operation. She and Peter resumed playing golf, a pastime they enjoyed!

8

Substance abuse and depression

➲ Key points

◆ Alcohol is very often used for self-medication against anxiety and depression.

◆ Changes in brain function as well as negative social repercussions cause depression amongst alcohol and drug abusers.

◆ Sometimes treatment of the actual addiction is enough to relieve depression. But the patient must be detoxified before any definite diagnosis of depressive illness is made.

◆ Tobacco affects the brain's chemical reward system thus depression may arise when a heavy smoker suddenly gives up smoking.

◆ As well as antidepressant medication, social support is important in the treatment of depression amongst substance abusers.

Some 20–30% of people suffering from mood disorders, i.e. depression or manic-depressive illness, misuse alcohol or are alcohol dependent. Alcohol and drugs should under no circumstances be used for self-medication; both depression and anxiety are exacerbated by dependence on, or addiction to, alcohol or drugs.

Alcohol, drug abuse, and depression

Alcohol is very often used for self-medication against anxiety and depression. When the short-lived effect of alcohol passes and sobriety returns even deeper depression and anguish are experienced. Alcoholics also develop tolerance, which means they have to drink on an increasing scale to dampen their anxiety and alleviate their depressive symptoms. The same applies to drugs: initially, drugs can relieve depressive symptoms, but in the long term they exacerbate the depression and anxiety. Substances classified as alcohol or narcotics should therefore under no circumstances be used for self-medication in depression.

Sometimes treatment of the actual addiction is enough to relieve depression. However, some substance abusers should be treated with antidepressant medication. It is important for the patient to be detoxified before any definite diagnosis of depressive illness is made.

Some investigations have shown that when alcoholics are treated with antide-pressants, not only their depression but also their craving for alcohol is reduced. The best results from treatment of depressed alcoholics are attained with antidepressant medication combined with psychosocial support. In the treatment of alcoholism, social support, such as that from Alcoholics Anonymous, is important.

Drug addicts, like alcoholics, may develop depressions both due to abuse and in conjunction with abstinence. Some studies have shown that, in drug addicts, antidepressants can both cure depression and prevent relapse into abuse.

Tobacco and depression

Tobacco is the addictive substance that, until now, has been most socially acceptable. As tobacco affects the brain's chemical reward system, including dopamine levels, depression may arise when a heavy smoker suddenly gives up smoking. There are people who smoke as an attempt to alleviate their depression. There is, in fact, no difference in abstinence patterns between tobacco and, for example, alcohol, morphine, and cocaine. Smokers who have been depressed previously, at one time or another in their lives, are those who run the greatest risk of relapse when they try to give up smoking.

📄 James, aged 44: depressed alcoholic

James owns a small food shop in south London. The shop is located near a school, and children usually come in to buy sweets. When James became the proprietor 15 years ago he thought it was fun that the schoolchildren came into his shop in the breaks. James used to chat to them, and heard quite a lot about their problems at school and at home.

Five years ago, James's eldest son was severely injured in a car accident. He is now confined to a wheelchair and will probably never walk again. A drunken motorist drove into him at a pedestrian crossing when he was on his way to school. A few months after the accident, James began to experience intense anguish. He began drinking alcohol to dampen it, but felt worse. He was dejected and had difficulty in falling asleep at night. He often woke up several times a night, and had nightmares about his son's car accident. Eventually, he started drinking in working hours.

He no longer chatted to the young people who came into the shop and was irritated with everyone. Everything felt hopeless, and James felt he had got stuck in a vicious circle. Finally, he did not even meet his friends. He withdrew from them, was deeply despondent, and felt that work was tedious. James began thinking of selling his shop, which he loved so much.

Although James's wife Jenny thought he should see a doctor for advice, he could not be bothered. It was nonsense, he thought. Once when James was in a period of drinking continuously and the shop was closed for several weeks, Jenny told him that he must either see the doctor or she would divorce him. James was shocked by these harsh words, but at the same time realized that she was probably right. The doctor prescribed a 'detox' for James. A few weeks after completing the detox James saw a psychiatrist who diagnosed him as depressed.

The doctor explained that antidepressants could be tried to treat the depression, although James did not believe they would help. James felt unwell on the medication and wanted to stop. He complained of impaired vision and a dry mouth, and he was constipated. The doctor persuaded him to put up with these side-effects. The depression lifted after a couple of months, and after another 2 months James's anxiety was also relieved.

James now has difficulty in remembering how his anguish and depression felt. As soon as he does not enjoy schoolchildren coming into his shop and picking at his sweets, he knows that the depression is returning. When he stops seeing his friends and feels a strong craving for the bottle, he knows it is time to visit the doctor. Despite his strong resistance to medicine he usually takes it regularly as, after a while, he feels more alert and can look after his shop again and joke with the youngsters.

For the past year James has also been receiving supportive psychotherapy. In this therapy he has learnt to deal with his anguish about his son's life situation. 'I never thought a few pills and a bit of talking could help anybody,' says James. 'But they did more for me than alcohol.'

9

Eating disturbances and depression

> ## ⊃ Key points
>
> ◆ In anorexia the compulsion to stop eating develops successively: starting with a desire to stop eating carbohydrates and escalating into rejection of all foods.
>
> ◆ Bulimics feel compelled to indiscriminately consume food and then promptly vomit.
>
> ◆ Both anorectics and bulimics:
>
>   ◆ Are fixated on their body weight and appearance.
>
>   ◆ Are unable to interpret their bodies' signals correctly.
>
>   ◆ Lose control of their bodies.
>
>   ◆ Are often depressed.
>
>   ◆ Find it difficult to resist the compulsive urge to starve or overeat.
>
>   ◆ Often abuse other substances and alcohol.
>
> ◆ Parents, teachers, family, and friends should pay attention as soon as they notice that girls or boys are starting to skip meals, limit their food intake, or avoid certain dishes.
>
> ◆ It is vital to seek psychological and medical treatment as soon as a person's eating disturbance becomes noticeable.

In the press and on the radio and television, the words 'anorexia' (self-starvation) and 'bulimia' (compulsive eating) crop up frequently. In magazines, one page may catalogue teenagers suffering from anorexia and bulimia while the next offers advice on the quickest and most effective slimming diet. This double message confuses many young girls and boys, making them anxious.

The teenage years

Teenagers should never embark on slimming diets, as they easily lose control over their own bodies. The ideals conveyed by the press and other media that a slender figure is desirable are reprehensible. The 'fashionable' image of the ideal woman being slim over the past decades has given a powerful boost to these food-related illnesses, and it will take time before this feminine ideal assumes reasonable proportions in our culture.

Mothers who are concerned about their figures and deliberately restrict their food intake should remember that this kind of attitude can influence their teenage daughters. In puberty and subsequently, for a few years, it is natural for young girls—owing to their hormonal development—to be a little chubby. This 'puppy fat' disappears naturally around the age of 20, or slightly later in young women. During the teenage years a balanced diet and proper exercise are extremely important, not only for the body, but are also necessary for the brain to develop normally.

Many children and teenagers, who try to lose weight and are concerned about what they should and should not eat, are discontented with their bodies. Young people with poor self-confidence believe that losing weight and becoming slim will enable them to attain happiness, success, and popularity. With these models and motives, it is hardly surprising that girls and boys start slimming and engage in hard physical training, and then succumb to either anorexia or bulimia.

It is very common for young girls who are anorexic to become depressed: the suicide rate is 20 times higher than in young people in general. New findings have shown that boys also suffer from anorexia and bulimia. Studies support a familial link between eating disorders.

Anorexia

In anorexia the compulsion to stop eating begins with a desire to stop eating carbohydrates, especially sweets, and escalates into rejection of all food containing fat. Eventually, the anorectic just picks at food. People with a food fixation commonly also start exercising a great deal, in many cases daily, and their food intake may decrease steadily by the day. Anorexic girls get thinner and thinner, and feel progressively worse, without managing to stop their compulsive behaviour. They lose control over their bodies and begin to resemble shadows of their former selves.

With anorexia, young girls' menstruation may stop and they develop digestive problems, such as constipation. With the disappearance of fat deposits, the young person's emaciated body becomes highly sensitive to cold. Although anorexics may look like skeletons, they can no longer perceive this; instead, they have distorted self-images of fat and shapeless bodies. Their judgment and view of reality are also disturbed.

Bulimia

Bulimics indiscriminately consume chocolate, crisps, cream, butter, fatty, and other foods out of an inner compulsion, and then promptly vomit. This kind of compulsive behaviour, with overeating and compulsive vomiting, may occur several times a week. Bulimics usually have corrosion damage on the back of their front teeth owing to the acid brought up from the stomach during vomiting. The bodies of bulimics become shapeless, commonly they put on a great deal of weight and, in girls, their menstrual periods may cease.

Bulimics and anorexics show some similarities. Both are fixated on their body weight and appearance, and unable to interpret their bodies' signals correctly. In both cases, they lose control of their bodies. Both anorexics and bulimics find it difficult to resist the compulsive urge to starve themselves or overeat. Abuse of alcohol, cannabis, and other drugs, and also certain asocial forms of behaviour such as shoplifting, are not unusual.

Treatment

Bulimia and anorexia occur mainly in girls and women. There are also some people who alternate between bulimia and anorexia. Depression is frequent. In the treatment of both anorexia and bulimia, it is firstly essential to stop the process of weight loss or compulsive eating, before the compulsive symptoms develop to the full. Behaviour and cognitive behaviour therapy methods combined with medication can be used.

Parents and teachers should pay attention and act as soon as they notice that girls or boys are starting to skip meals, limit their food intake, or avoid certain dishes. Enjoyable mealtime rituals may, in time, offset negative behaviour in children and young people who start dieting. When the slimming or overeating process has progressed too far, parents are often helpless and the situation is beyond their control. It is therefore vital to seek psychological and medical treatment as soon as a child's eating disturbance becomes noticeable.

10

Anxiety and depression

⮕ Key points

❖ The risk of succumbing to a state of anxiety at one time or another in one's life is about 20–25% for women and 10% for men.

❖ The common anxiety disorders are: generalized anxiety disorder (GAD), panic disorder, phobias, social phobia, and obsessive–compulsive disorders (OCD).

❖ Rational anxiety is a natural response to life crises such as life-threatening situations or disasters.

❖ Irrational anxiety occurs without a clear cause and often presents itself in an exaggerated, extraordinary reaction to ordinary events.

❖ Panic disorder is the sudden onset of acute anxiety. These anxiety attacks or 'panic attacks' can occur regularly or sporadically.

❖ Anxiety, like depression, can be treated by both medication and psychological treatments. A stable and calm environment also helps to settle those with a predisposition towards anxiety.

It is common for depressed people also to suffer from anxiety and its extreme form, anguish. However, anxiety may sometimes mask depression and in such cases sufferers do not realize that they are depressed.

Symptoms of anxiety

The anguish I experienced during a depression was a terrifying feeling I was unable to shake off.

A patient

The psychological symptoms of anxiety are:

- A strong feeling of apprehension and fear

- Inner tension

- Difficulty in concentrating

- Irritability

- Increased hypersensitivity to noise

- Sleep disturbances.

Common physical symptoms might be:

- Increased muscular tension

- Severe headaches

- Tension throughout the body

- Heart palpitations or chest pain

- Shortness of breath and hyperventilation

- Stomach pain

- Diarrhoea

- Mouth dryness

- Marked reduction in libido

- Buzzing in the ears

- Dizziness

- A tingling sensation in the extremities.

Worry, restlessness, and anguish are also common symptoms of all types of depression in both children and adults. An estimated 60% of depressed people suffer from severe anxiety states.

Although it is sometimes difficult to distinguish between depression and anxiety, the essential difference is that depression is characterized by inhibition, whereas anxiety involves agitation. A feeling of pointlessness and hopelessness are symptoms that characterize depression but are absent in anxiety disorders, in which more physical symptoms and phobias occur.

Types of anxiety

Anxiety may be a signal that something in a person's life situation is unsatisfactory. This type is often called 'signal anxiety', and the signal may spur people to tackle their problems, change their situation, and develop. But when sufferers are, owing to their biological and psychological susceptibility, unable to deal with a difficult life situation, their anxiety may become intense, persistent, and terrible.

There is often a blurred line between what is called rational or justified anxiety and irrational or 'pathological' anxiety. Rational anxiety is a natural reaction to life crises, life-threatening situations, or disasters, such as wars, terrorist attacks, and earthquakes. Irrational anxiety or anguish may arise without a person really knowing why, or as a magnified reaction to ordinary events that should not provoke such a state.

Anxiety disorders and depression

All anxiety states described below may coincide with various depressive conditions.

Generalized anxiety disorder (GAD)

In GAD the anxiety is not intense, but it is constant. This type of anxiety is hard to control, and is always present in combination with an exaggerated apprehension at the prospect of forthcoming activities or events. The sufferer is often anxious and worried about entirely insignificant matters. Besides worry, people suffer from a range of other symptoms, such as fatigue, muscular tension, restlessness, and irritation. They feel heavy-headed, have difficulty in falling asleep, and wake easily. The anguish increases with stress and, if the stress is severe, depression may develop.

Post-traumatic stress disorder

A combination of anxiety and depression may also ensue from traumatic experiences, in which case the condition is known as 'post-traumatic stress disorder' (PTSD). Examples of the kinds of events that can cause PTSD are air crashes, shipwrecks, wars, terrorist attacks, and natural disasters.

Cognitive behavioural therapy (CBT), behavioural therapy, and antidepressants are relevant in the treatment of PTSD. Symptoms may be alleviated by various forms of repeated exposure to situations that caused the PTSD.

Panic attacks

Panic disorder is characterized by the sudden onset of anxiety in highly acute attacks. These attacks may come several times daily or just occasionally once a month or year. In an attack, the anxiety escalates from tension, with acute apprehension, to a sense of doom and panic with total loss of self-control. Accompanying the panic are physical symptoms: chest pain, cardiac palpitations, and a rapid pulse. Victims may become short of breath, have the sensation of choking, and feel that they are on the verge of death. Nausea, stomach pain, vertigo, and shivering are other common symptoms. The panic attack often ceases after a few minutes, but may sometimes go on for hours.

A person who has experienced a panic attack is exhausted, and falls prey to a new fear: that of the next attack. This fear is itself a form of anxiety known as 'anticipatory anxiety'. Fear of recurrent attacks may result in phobic behaviour, such as agoraphobia or claustrophobia. These phobic types of behaviour afford protection, enabling the person to avoid situations that provoke attacks.

Specific phobias

The most common anxiety syndromes, which appear in approximately 10% of the population sometime during their lives, are specific phobias. Specific phobia is characterized by irrational fear in very special situations like for example, treatment at the dentist, flights, high places, exposure to blood, spiders, or snakes. Usually this kind of phobia does place restrictions on everyday life; however, in some cases it can cause a significant handicap.

Agoraphobia and claustrophobia

Agoraphobia means fear not of the *agora* (Greek for 'marketplace'; the word is used to mean all wide open spaces) itself, but of being unable to escape from a crowd. People often do not fear crowds as such, but rather the throng that would prevent them from obtaining help if they suffered an attack in a public place. Agoraphobia is found in roughly 0.5–1% of the population, mainly women.

In claustrophobia, the panic attack arises in situations that involve restriction of movement, such as going in a lift, sitting in a dentist's chair, travelling by train through a tunnel, being on board an aircraft. Claustrophobia is exacerbated by darkness.

Agoraphobia and claustrophobia may sometimes mask depression, and both states may occur with or without panic disorder. Effects of antidepressants are limited. Cognitive behavioural therapy (CBT) and behavioural therapy, with exposure to situations that evoke fear, may alleviate mild and moderate types of phobia.

Social phobia

Social phobia means that one experiences fear and anxiety at the prospect of meeting unknown people. The reason may be that one feels inferior to others. It is often shy people and those with poor self-confidence who suffer from social phobia. This kind of phobia is common in the depressed. In those with major depression, social phobia is found in 24–28% of cases. In sufferers from manic-depressive illness social phobia may be present.

In social phobia, as in depression, self-medication with alcohol and drugs is common. This is dangerous, because addiction may develop. As tolerance increases, the individual must constantly raise the dose to attain a soothing or mood-enhancing effect. Alcohol and illicit drugs make both depression and anxiety worse in the long run. Under no circumstances, therefore, should alcohol or illicit drugs be used for self-medication in social phobias or depressions.

Obsessive–compulsive disorder (OCD)

In OCD, the anxiety is related to obsessional thoughts or compulsive rituals that oblige a person to think or act in a particular way to avoid anxiety or anguish. Both obsessive thoughts and compulsive actions are involuntary, i.e. cannot be controlled by sheer willpower. Examples of obsessive thoughts are recurrent brooding about the same matters and fear of losing self-control, for example killing a family member or laughing at a funeral. Examples of compulsive acts are checking over and over again that the oven is switched off, or the door is locked. Obsessive and compulsive symptoms may be the first signs of profound depression in manic-depressive illness or schizophrenia.

Treatment of depression-related anxiety

In the treatment of anxiety, as in that of depression, both medication and various forms of psychological treatments may be effective. Exposure to the situations and stimuli that evoke anxiety is often highly beneficial.

Antidepressants and sedatives

In the treatment of severe anxiety with antidepressant drugs, it takes several weeks—sometimes several months—before relief arises and the symptoms of anguish abate. Antidepressants are not deemed to be habit-forming, and therefore constitute an important treatment tool, but often need to be combined with sedatives initially in the treatment of anxiety. Depression is alleviated much more rapidly than anxiety in treatment with antidepressants, and results are often attained after 4–6 weeks.

Psychological forms of treatment

When antidepressants begin to work the anxiety is bearable, but seldom disappears entirely. The reason is that anxiety or anguish often has psychological causes, and psychological help is therefore necessary to understand and learn how to cope with it. The various forms of psychological treatment used in care of the depressed, like CBT, behavioural therapy, and psychodynamic therapy are described in Chapter 19, and show good effects on anxiety.

Treatment of anxiety in children and adolescents

In children and adolescents, treatment with antidepressants alone is recommended only in severe OCD. In other conditions, behavioural therapy, with or without cognitive components is recommended. A combination of antidepressants and behavioural therapy or CBT seems to reinforce the positive effects.

Combination treatment

A combination of psychological treatment and antidepressant medication is very often used in recurrent and long-lasting depressions with bouts of anxiety. Combined treatments are particularly recommended for people suffering from anxiety and depression when the risk of suicidal acts is elevated, and also in chronic conditions.

11

Sleep and depression

> ## ⟳ Key points
>
> ◆ Sleep takes up a third of our life and allows our body to release tension and recover from the stresses of daily life.
>
> ◆ Short term sleep deficiency is not harmful; however regularly having less than 5 hours sleep per night can negatively affect an adult's health.
>
> ◆ Long term sleep deficiency increases the risk of heart and digestive disorders, as well as depression.
>
> ◆ Catnapping is a good and effective way of making up for lost sleep. Even a 15 minute nap sitting in a chair boosts energy and concentration.
>
> ◆ Regular bed times, a cool dark bedroom with a comfortable bed, peace and quiet, and avoidance of caffeine, nicotine, and alcohol in the evening (or several hours before), can all assist a good sleep.
>
> Some deeply despondent people sleep more than usual, but the great majority of depressed people sleep less than usual. They may also have difficulty in falling asleep, and then wake up in the small hours, tossing and turning in their beds.

Normal sleep

Sleep takes up a third of our lives. During sleep our breathing slows down, and blood pressure, pulse, metabolism, and body temperature all fall whilst muscular tensions decrease and the central nervous system gets a chance to recover. Children and young people who are growing need a great deal of deep sleep. Adults, on average, need 7 ½ hours' sleep a night. The minimum

Sleep stages

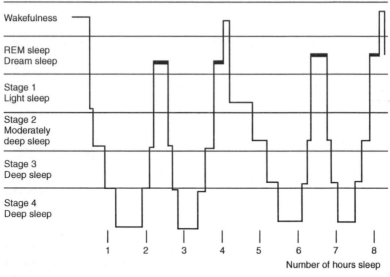

Figure 11.1 Normal sleep cycle in a non-depressed person.

amount appears to be 5–6 hours. Short-term sleep deficiencies have hardly any bearing on our health. Sleep requirements are, however, highly individual and vary from one person to another.

Sleep consists of various stages, which form a cycle (see Figure 11.1). During the night there are four or five sleep cycles, which in healthy people form a fairly constant pattern. A normal night's sleep consists of two different types of sleep: the stable form divided into four stages and a stage of dream sleep (rapid eye movement, REM sleep). On falling asleep, we pass through a stage of light sleep. This is a transition between a waking state and sleep, and in this stage, people are easily woken. For this reason, silence is important when trying to fall asleep. People who suffer from brief or chronic depression are easily roused.

After the first stage, sleep enters stage 2 of moderately deep sleep, called consolidated sleep. Stages 3 and 4 consist of deep sleep in which maximum recovery of brain functions takes place. After just over an hour's sleep we return to stage 2 and then to stage 1 again, where a stage of dream sleep 'REM sleep', lasting for 5–20 minutes, begins.

The more our emotions are affected when we are awake, owing to pleasant or unpleasant events, the more lively our dreams become. A person who, for example, has been under heavy pressure during the day tends to have nightmares, as dreams contain fragments connected with what has happened previously.

We have vivid dreams during REM sleep, and if we are woken up during these periods we usually remember our dreams. The last REM period of the night is the most intense. We dream roughly four to five times a night during the REM stage. Researchers believe that it is in REM sleep that we work out solutions to our problems.

Duration of sleep

Sleep changes with age. Newborn babies sleep about 16–18 hours a day, and 50% of this sleep is REM sleep. An adult usually needs 7–8 hours, of which 6 hours constitute stable sleep and one and a half hours are REM sleep. The elderly sleep less and wake frequently. If we wake up for less than 2 minutes, we are unaware of doing so.

Sleep and wakefulness are regulated by our daily rhythm, which depends on alternation between darkness and light. Our biological clock is brought forward by early morning light and set back by late light in the evenings. This is why our rhythm changes during the year.

Neurons and neural pathways—especially in the brainstem—are involved in sleep regulation by a hormone called melatonin. Secretion of melatonin is governed by the rhythmic alternation of light and darkness, through neural pathways leading from the eye to the brain. Its production decreases with advancing age. Melatonin enhances the sensitivity of the brain's receptors that regulate our emotions.

If normal length of sleep is reduced, we are tired, attention and learning capacity are impaired, and we function poorly. A short-term sleep deficiency can be made up on the following night: as we fall asleep more rapidly and slumber more deeply. It is therefore unnecessary to sleep longer on the following night in order to compensate for a shortage of sleep.

Prolonged sleep deficiency, e.g. because of late night shifts, work in shifts, early morning work, or care of dependents, all have negative health effects. The risk for cardiovascular diseases and gastrointestinal diseases increases.

Catnaps

Catnapping is a good and effective way of making up for lost sleep. A nap can last from 15 minutes to an hour, depending on how easily one falls asleep.

Feeling tired or sleepy, or finding it difficult to concentrate, is a good reason for having a short sleep in a comfortable bed or on the sofa. Many people also benefit from a short nap that may be taken seated in an armchair, during a working day. There is a striking increase in work capacity and attention after a rest of this kind.

One sleeps best between midnight and eight o'clock in the morning. One should preferably avoid getting up before six o'clock in the morning. Loss of sleep due to early rising is hard to make up for by going to bed earlier; instead, try a nap during the day.

Sleep patterns in the depressed

Insomnia is a constant problem in 8% and perhaps up to 10% of the population, especially in the middle-aged and elderly. Sleep problems are frequent in depression but also in conjunction with pain, physical illnesses, and personal problems. However, sleep needs are individual and most people sleep more than they think.

Two important characteristics—length of time taken to fall asleep and continuity—denote sleep quality. In the depressed, patterns of falling asleep and sleep continuity are in sharp contrast to those in healthy people. 75% of depressed people suffer from insomnia, i.e. have difficulty in falling asleep, their thoughts keep grinding round in their heads about current or previous problems. Sleep is superficial, with many interruptions and sleep continuity is poor as they wake up and cannot settle. Brooding thoughts are oppressive. Nightmares are common in despondent individuals, especially those suffering from melancholia. Depressed people wake up early in the morning, having had little deep sleep, which is very important for recuperation. This is why despondent people do not feel fully rested in the morning.

Antidepressant medication and sleep

Antidepressant medication, as well as lithium and electroconvulsive therapy, usually normalize depressed people's sleep patterns. The medication extends the period from falling asleep to the commencement of REM sleep. Total REM sleep, of which depressed people have far too much, is reduced.

Melatonin

Elderly people who have problems in falling asleep often have low melatonin levels. Treatment with melatonin tablets to tackle sleep problems in the elderly, and sleep disturbances due to jet lag, is recommended. Blind people with disruptions in their daily rhythm, and accompanying sleep problems, are a group for which melatonin can be prescribed.

Simple self-help measures to improve sleep

Depressed people should stick to regular times for going to bed and getting up. If sleep refuses to come one should not keep looking at the clock. It is better, instead, to get up and go to another room, and spend some time there, preferably engaged in some monotonous activity. The second room should be slightly warmer than the bedroom. This sensation of warmth can help drowsiness, making it easier to fall asleep later in the cool bedroom.

The bedroom should be dark with a cool temperature of 15–18° Celsius and painted in soothing pastel colours. Before going to bed, open the windows to let fresh air in. A comfortable bed, with pillows and a duvet of good quality, is a must. Cool, clean sheets, improve sleep quality.

One should try to eliminate the risk of being woken up by noise or other disturbances. A snoring partner should be assisted to stop, and earplugs used to block out disturbing noises. Adults and children suffering from anxiety sleep better with a night-light switched on.

It is a good idea to have a transition period before going to bed. One can, for example, take a short walk, as moderate physical activity improves sleep. Various relaxation techniques are also helpful in ensuring good sleep. Relaxing in a hot bath, listening to soothing music, and drinking hot milk may help. Do not go to sleep hungry. An excess intake of alcohol in the evening, does, it is true, hasten the onset of sleep but makes sleep superficial.

Nicotine has a stimulating effect and can disturb sleep, as can caffeine. For 5–7 hours before going to bed, avoid beverages containing caffeine, such as coffee, tea, and Coca Cola. Caffeine has a stimulating effect, and is also a diuretic, thus waking up more frequently due to the need to urinate.

PART 2

Causes of depression

12

Biological theories on the causes of depression

> ## ⮕ Key points
>
> ◆ Neurotransmitters in the brain regulate motor activity, help learning, memory capacity, and emotional processing.
>
> ◆ The main neurotransmitters associated with depression and anxiety are: serotonin, dopamine, and noradrenaline.
>
> ◆ Serotonin affects body temperature, regulation of sleep and wakefulness, mood regulation and impulse control.
>
> ◆ Noradrenaline helps in regulating mood and anxiety levels.
>
> ◆ Dopamine regulates motor and mental activity, attention and motivation.
>
> The interaction and balance between neurotransmitters plays an important part in mood regulation and the emergence of affective illnesses i.e. those relating to emotions.

The brain's neurotransmitters and regulation of the emotions

The brain contains up to 100 billion neurons. Communication between neurons takes place through special sites of contact known as synapses, which are located on the nerve ends. The messages transmitted between neurons are conveyed by amines or amino acids that are neurotransmitters. Our emotional life is affected by the function of the various neurotransmitters and the interaction between them. The main neurotransmitters cited frequently in connection with depression and anxiety are serotonin, dopamine, and noradrenaline.

Serotonin and depression

Serotonin is known to affect body temperature, regulation of sleep and wakefulness, hormone secretion, and food intake. Besides mood regulation, serotonin is also involved in perception of external stimuli and impulse control. Imbalance in the serotonin system may provoke depression and panic anxiety, as well as aggressive behaviour and obsessive-compulsive symptoms.

Personality traits that are hereditary as well as environmentally conditioned appear to depend, to some extent, on serotonin functioning. People with high serotonin levels have been shown to be confident, optimistic, relaxed, and neither aggressive nor impulsive. They are also self-critical and conscientious. People with low serotonin levels, on the other hand, are aggressive, competitive, and more impulsive, but may also be fearful and inhibited.

Noradrenaline and depression

Noradrenaline is another neurotransmitter that plays a part in regulating mood and anxiety level. The view that both acute and chronic stress may result in depression is generally accepted. The noradrenaline cells are highly active in situations that call for alert attention and readiness for self-defence, partly by controlling circulation and breathing. Moreover, noradrenaline is involved in analysis of the information received by the brain from various sensory organs, such as the eye.

Dopamine and depression

Dopamine is a neurotransmitter that plays a part in initiating motor and mental activity, and is thought to be involved in the emergence of depressive illnesses. Dopamine also regulates mental processes, which are connected with attention and motivation. In Parkinson's disease dopamine levels are low, and in certain psychoses dopamine activity is excessively high.

Dopamine levels and dopamine activity also affects personality traits. Low dopaminergic activity may result in difficulty feeling joy and pleasure in life. At the same time, people with low dopamine levels are relatively analytical and stable, and do not readily break up relationships. People with high dopamine levels, on the other hand, are impulsive, seek excitement and take decisions on the spur of the moment; change partner, job, and interests frequently; and may be self-destructive.

Melatonin and depression

Melatonin is a hormone that exhibits connections with depression. Production of melatonin is governed by light and dark. The melatonin system is part of our biological clock and regulates our daily rhythm of wakefulness and sleep. In healthy people, the maximum level of melatonin is observed between 2 and 4 o'clock in the morning. In depressed people, and especially those suffering from melancholia, melatonin levels are evened out. On recovery from depression, melatonin levels return to the normal pattern—highest at night and lowest in the morning.

Prolactin and depression

Prolactin is another hormone that affects our mental state. This hormone stimulates milk production in nursing mothers, but is also found in men. In depression that is characterized by apathy, weight gain, and reduced libido, prolactin levels in both men and women may be elevated. People with poor self-esteem and weak social support who simultaneously experience a feeling of powerlessness very often have high prolactin levels. This applies to men and women alike.

The immune system and mental well-being

The immune system is the body's defence reaction against infection, but also rejects certain tumour cells and interacts closely with the central nervous system. It has long been known that during depression and stress, especially chronic stress, the body's immune defence mechanisms are weakened. Research shows that deeply depressed people who have attempted suicide have reduced activity in various cells of the immune system, and this may be due to a prolonged state of stress. It is also well known that the incidence of certain infections, such as herpes (mouth or genital ulcers) increases at times of stress.

Depression and diseases in hormone-producing organs

Stress and illnesses with direct effects on hormone-producing organs also affect the secretion of hormones, which in turn disturb hormonal balance and may lead to depression. In the event of, in particular, a deficiency of thyroxine, which is produced in the thyroid gland, some people become despondent and anxious. The most salient symptoms, however, are usually fatigue and a marked impairment in cognitive functions. Treatment of depression associated with thyroxine deficiency consists primarily in supplying thyroid hormone in tablet form. As a secondary measure, antidepressants are prescribed.

13

Psychological theories of depression

→ Key points

- Physical and emotional changes affect the central nervous system and can negatively influence psychological functioning.

- The 'biopsychosocial' model shows that a depressed person's individual experiences, combined with biological, social, and environmental factors, are what cause depression.

- Cognitive theories focus on adverse life conditions or stress, dysfunctional attitudes, and beliefs that can induce depression.

- Lack of supportive networks, poorly functioning relationships, and poor social integration are associated with an increased risk of depression.

- Some types of personality disorder are linked to depression and anxiety and should be considered in the assessment of depression.

Psychological theories deal with issues of perception, appraisal, and belief formation, and touch on the psychological elements of everyday life, such as love, duties, and achievements. Depressive states require a psychological approach: they cannot be explained solely in terms of brain function.

Biopsychosocial model

The biopsychosocial model assumes that a depressed person's individual experiences, combined with biological, social, and environmental factors, are what bring about depression. Research shows that depressed people are helped not only by biological treatment that changes chemical processes in the brain, but also by psychological treatments and approaches in which experiential factors are addressed.

Cognitive model of depression

Depression, when activated by adverse life conditions and stress, is associated with dysfunctional attitudes and beliefs. In anxiety disorder, depression, and other mental disorders, thoughts that recall negative life events of childhood are often observed. Cognitive behavioural therapy helps people to focus on problem-solving strategies and develop their ability to modify their depressive beliefs and attitudes.

Social theory of depression and learned helplessness

A state of so-called learned helplessness is a reaction to adverse life experiences and socially disadvantageous environments, such as lack of supportive networks, poorly functioning relationships with parents, partner, family and friends, and poor social integration. Living in conditions of social deprivation and poverty, or in an environment that is disadvantageous in other ways, may evoke feelings of hopelessness.

When parental role models do not demonstrate how to deal with these conditions and there is emotional deprivation, a sense of helplessness may arise with the realization that very little or nothing can be done to improve or change one's life situation. Depression can be a direct consequence of the psychological perception that there is no point trying to do anything. Perceptions of this kind can prompt not only depression and anxiety, but also criminal or other antisocial activities.

Developmental model of depression and the role of negative life events

Children's relationships with their parents have a bearing on their emotions and behaviour throughout life. Deprivation of parental care due to separation from parents, owing to divorce or other marital problems is a factor found to cause elevated depression rates. Emotional, physical, and sexual abuse affects the child's emotions and cognition and governs their actions and relationships with others. Depression, anxiety, or other mental health problems occur, according to psychodynamic theories, when a conflict from an early experience is activated in adult life.

Parents of depressed children often have their own history of depression. This may be reflected in ineffective communication, resulting in poor parent–child interactions and alienation from the family, which is the most important source of support and social bonding. The adverse impact of early negative life events and risk factors may continue to have a negative influence during adolescence, especially if high-risk children live in an unstable context, without support.

Protective factors

Protective factors, such as sustained prevention and treatment activities that afford stronger support for the child and parents alike can counteract negative development. Encouraging positive involvement with parents and non-depressed peers is one remedy. Teaching children problem-solving and emotional coping skills is another. These methods help to boost children's self-esteem, helping to prevent them from lapsing into a depressive state.

Personality types predisposed to depression

For people with certain personality features, the risk of incurring depression is relatively high. However, not everyone with the traits mentioned below necessarily becomes depressed. Whether a person with a particular personality type develops depression depends both on inheritance and environment.

- **People of an asthenic disposition** are tense, uncertain, shy, and easily exhausted. Conscientious, but susceptible to stress, they find it difficult to make decisions and assert themselves. Lacking confidence in their own ability, they avoid confrontations and conflicts. They do not venture to take the initiative socially, or enjoy what life can offer. Very often, they are excessively cautious and afraid of failure or disappointment. Asthenics may withdraw socially, isolating themselves, because of shyness which contributes to the development of depression.

- **People of a pessimistic disposition** interpret the surrounding world negatively. Exaggerated pessimism is often observed in people who suffer from 'persistent depression' (dysthymia). Dysthymics feel constantly dissatisfied and irritated. Their attitude towards others may be demanding, as they constantly feel that other people lack understanding of their needs. Dysthymics have difficulty in enjoying life, their families, and their own success.

- **People of a compulsive disposition who are pedantic and intolerant** may succumb to depression. Individuals of a compulsive nature may incur depression when away from work, due to a lack of routine. They usually feel best when they are engaged in work involving strict routines. People with exaggerated compulsive features may become isolated, as others are frustrated by their manner. This social isolation may, in turn, result in depression.

◆ **People of a narcissistic disposition** have a great need to be seen, appreciated, and admired. Divorce, criticism, or lack of promotion may be perceived by a narcissistically inclined person as deeply wounding, and depression may result. The risk of depression increases with age, when narcissistic people lose their youthful appearance and vigour.

◆ **People of a cyclothymic disposition** have mood-swings which alternate between a sense of well-being and despondency. Cyclothymics often impose high demands on themselves. They are often charming, warm, cordial, empathetic, open, and easy-going. Some cyclothymics may push themselves hard to do far too much for other people out of a fear of not being needed. This behaviour drains their mental and physical strength, and causes them to neglect their own needs. As cyclothymics' mission in life is to look after and help others, they are vulnerable to criticism.

◆ **People of an impulsive disposition** are easily carried away by their feelings and overreact to setbacks. They have difficulty in exerting control over themselves, and easily become frustrated when those around them disapprove of their impulsive actions.

14

Nature or nurture: what matters most?

> ### 🔁 Key points
>
> ◆ Adrenaline and cortisol are the known 'stress-hormones'.
>
> ◆ In prolonged stress, not only do mental symptoms such as anguish and depression develop but physical symptoms also arise and the immune system is affected.
>
> ◆ A person's nature (inherited biological traits) and nurture (environment) are very closely interwoven and must both be taken into consideration when treating depression.
>
> The complex interaction between nature (heredity) and nurture (environment) explains the causes and course of depressive illnesses. Hereditary disposition and acquired hypersensitivity due to trauma in early life have a bearing on how the body's psycho-neuro-hormonal system copes with mental and social stress and whether depression develops.

The stress-vulnerability model

For a long time, two different models explaining depression—one focusing on inborn biological characteristics regulated by genes and the other underlining the significance of mental and social trauma—have coexisted in separate worlds. Modern depression research, however, takes into consideration the close links between these two models, and follows the stress-vulnerability model.

Biological endowment

Children that receive inadequate parental care or chronic stress may develop undesirable changes in the functioning and interaction of the central nervous system and the hormonal systems. This may be why children who are exposed to separation and traumatic events as they are growing up react to stress situations in adulthood not only psychologically, but also biologically.

Human temperament and reactions depend on our genetic makeup, but our personality and identity development are also influenced by the environment we live in. Temperament is sharpened and developed through social intercourse and by our upbringing. If a family's mental and social wellbeing is unsatisfactory, this may be compensated for by the child's social network in and out of school. If there are good examples in children's and young people's surroundings, they can learn to cope with their situation. Studies on twins have shown that in environments that lack psychosocial support, the risk of major depression increases.

Stress and depression

Today, we know that the balance between various neurotransmitters serves as the foundation for normal brain functioning and, accordingly, for our mental health. We also know that stress, both acute and chronic, stemming from recurrent strains in life brings about an elevated noradrenergic response and hypersensitivity of the noradrenaline receptors, in turn affecting both the dopamine and the serotonin system and resulting in an imbalance between various neurotransmitters in the brain. There is also research showing that certain brain cells may shrink as a result of severe traumatic experiences, thus brain functions are affected.

Cortisol stimulates the hippocampus, the part of the brain responsible for learning and memory. A surplus of cortisol can, however, have a toxic effect and lead to a reduction of cognitive functions. High concentrations of cortisol can lead to long-term changes. Increased sensitivity to cortisol due to renewed stress is characteristic of people who have previously experienced prolonged mental, physical, or social trauma.

Acute or chronic stress during childhood, under-stimulation and inadequate parent–child relationships, lack of positive models among family and associates, inadequate conflict resolution, a negative emotional climate, and destructive social circumstances can all lead to depression. Infections, toxic substances, alcohol and drug abuse, dietary deficiencies, and other physical factors that affect brain development at the foetal stage and childhood, are examples of environmental factors with an impact on the incidence of depression.

Our ways of dealing with our biological and psychosocial endowment and environmental factors depend on culture, education, social networks, and financial circumstances. Psychological and economic deprivation in low-income settings severely impairs children's biological and emotional development. However, our psychosocial and physical environment is something we can change, and this enables us to ward off depression and mental ill-health.

In prolonged stress, not only do mental symptoms such as anguish and depression develop but physical symptoms also arise. In individuals exposed to prolonged stress a range of different biological reactions, such as energy levels and the immune system, may be disturbed if stress recurs. Stressed people are more prone to infections, muscular aches, and the like. Even memories of former stress situations, such as previous torture, separations, and other traumas, may cause a person to react with both physical symptoms and mental ones such as anguish or depression.

PART 3

Treatment of depression

15

When to see a doctor and subsequent treatment

Key points

◆ When seeking medical help for depression, the following information is vital:

    ◆ Information about the course of the illness

    ◆ Prior depression

    ◆ Family medical history

    ◆ Other health concerns

    ◆ Social situation and network.

◆ Antidepressants stabilize a person's mood by restoring the balance between various neurotransmitters in the central nervous system.

◆ Psychological treatment for depression can help to improve self-esteem and promote flexible thinking: particularly for first-time sufferers, pregnant women, and young people.

◆ Prior to treatment for depression, people should ask their doctor:

    ◆ What type of depression they are suffering from

    ◆ What treatment options are available

    ◆ What the reasons are for trying a particular treatment

> ◆ What the advantages and disadvantages are
>
> ◆ If long-term preventative treatment is recommended.
>
> When a depressed person consults a medical professional, the doctor should weigh up the pros and cons of various treatment options choosing the one best suited to the person's unique situation and needs.

A human lifetime
spans less than a century,
but has a thousand sorrows:
the days are fleeting
and the nights bitterly long.
Why not take the lantern
and set out on a search?

Chinese wisdom from the Han Dynasty

When should one consult a doctor for treatment?

People who feel unwell or low-spirited, have difficulty in sleeping or being cheerful, notice that their work and social capacity are impaired, and that they are functioning poorly should see a doctor to obtain help in assessing whether they are depressed or merely despondent. Individuals suffering from a severe depression such as melancholia, or with psychotic symptoms—that is, individuals who depart entirely from their usual ways of functioning—should seek help without delay.

People with depression in the family run a risk of developing a depression themselves when, for example, they experience stress. They should recognize how well they feel, and seek help if they notice signs of depression. Sometimes they may need psychotherapy for preventive purposes, to learn how to deal with acute and chronic stress, which can lead to depression.

Information about the course of the illness and the individual as well as family medical and psychiatric history of prior depressive episodes is equally important, as is awareness that depression may have many different causes. This is why it is essential to identify environmental factors that affect its onset and course, so that the choice of treatment does not become a matter of routine.

Unfortunately, both depressed people and their relatives usually hesitate to contact a doctor. They may not, perhaps, believe that they suffer from an illness or that there are any treatment options that can help them. But this is wrong: good treatment methods exist for most depressive illnesses.

The doctor's considerations

Recovery from a depression is unique for every person. Prompt alleviation of depressive symptoms can usually be achieved with antidepressants, but it is not certain that medication alone can prevent relapses and a chronic course of depression. In many cases psychological treatment or advanced psychotherapy is necessary to enable depressed people to regain control over their own lives.

Different methods of treating depression vary in the rapidity with which symptoms are relieved and the depression lifts. It is also common for people, when starting treatment with antidepressants, to feel worse at first, however this deterioration is temporary. Side-effects usually diminish and are less troublesome after treatment has continued for some time.

Various forms of psychological treatment are as effective as treatment with antidepressants in mild and certain moderately severe forms of depression. However, it takes longer for the depressive symptoms and anguish to be relieved than in treatment with antidepressants. When it comes to preventing relapses, it seems important not only to undergo longterm treatment with antidepressants, but also for them to be combined with psychological treatment. Of depressed people who receive combination treatment (both antidepressants and psychological treatment simultaneously) 80–85% become symptom-free.

When should a psychiatrist be in charge of the treatment?

Antidepressant treatment of uncomplicated depression can be administered by a general practitioner. But even if non-specialists can diagnose the type of depression from which a person is suffering, a supplementary psychiatric or psychological specialist assessment may be called for, to ascertain the most appropriate type of treatment for a particular person.

In severe cases, treatment should be managed by a specialist in psychiatry. This applies, above all, to cases in which the people have serious and enduring thoughts of suicide and have attempted it, and also to depressions associated with other mental illnesses such as schizophrenia. Treatment of manic-depressive illness, hypomania, and substance abuse, and also depression connected with pregnancy or childbirth, should also be administered by a psychiatrist.

Treatment of depression in children and teenagers must always be under the supervision of a specialist in child and adolescent psychiatry.

Contact with relatives

Relatives are an important source of support for depressed people and they can obtain advice from a doctor, social worker, or psychologist as to how they can help the depressed person and understand the process they are going through.

As a person or a person's relative, one should never be afraid of asking the doctor questions. However, it is the depressed person who, in cooperation with the doctor, should arrive at the treatment option that is most suitable, with reference not only to the symptoms but also to personality, lifestyle, and general functioning.

Personality and treatment success

Before embarking on treatment for depression, people should ask their doctor what type of depression they are suffering from, what treatment options are available, and what reasons the doctor has for suggesting a particular treatment. The more thoroughly people are prepared for the advantages and disadvantages of a treatment method, the greater their chances are that the treatment will be successful. Even if the doctor considers that drug treatment would be best, a person's negative attitude towards medication may jeopardize its effects.

When is antidepressant treatment recommended?

Many people worry about using antidepressants; but they are not considered addictive, and offer relatively rapid recovery. Treatment with antidepressants affords freedom from symptoms in up to 70–75% of cases.

In the first place, antidepressants are recommended in the treatment of moderate and severe depressions, especially melancholias. People of a compulsive disposition who are depressed also respond well to antidepressants. When physical symptoms such as lack of appetite, weight loss, sleeplessness, and motor fatigue are troublesome, antidepressants are usually recommended for milder depressions as well.

Mildly depressed people who feel no need to explore their inner experience in depth and wish to be relieved of their symptoms as promptly as possible should also be recommended treatment with antidepressants. The offer of psychological treatment may be perceived as offensive, just as people who are interested in the existential questions of life may perceive an offer of medical treatment as an unsubtle way of dealing with their problem.

Medication is chosen with reference to the antidepressant effect and how rapidly this effect is desired. Certain people are prepared to wait longer for the antidepressant to take effect. Others may, perhaps, want a 'quick fix', and a fast-acting preparation that perhaps has more side-effects must then be prescribed. Doctors also take into consideration people's occupation and workload, in order to avoid side-effects that rule out the pursuit of their occupations. The doctor should also take into account whether the person has any other physical illnesses and must choose the kind of antidepressant that does not interact with other medication the person is taking.

Many depressed people find the side-effects of antidepressants troublesome, and discontinue their treatment before regaining their health. This is a pity, as the side-effects usually pass, and there are also several ways of counteracting them. In addition, the newer antidepressants have less troublesome side-effects.

When depressed people regain their health, both their sleeping patterns and their appetite improve. They look less tired, their memory and concentration capacity are better, and their vitality and willpower return. The pessimism disappears, and everything starts to feel more vibrant. Curiosity is aroused, and the cognitive functions improve. So, too, does their capacity to experience pleasure and joy. Their jobs seem interesting again, and they stop being tormented by brooding about what is right and wrong. Their work capacity expands. They feel more organized and settled.

'Happy pills'

Sometimes, owing to the extensive advertising of certain antidepressants, people expect their personalities to undergo sweeping changes, and think they will become carefree after a course of treatment. They anticipate a miracle, and believe that everything they have been unable to attain will happen after a few months' treatment with 'happy pills'. This is misleading. Antidepressants do not make people happy, but they help depressed people to become better or recover entirely.

When is electroconvulsive therapy (ECT) recommended?

In very severe depressions of a melancholic nature; with reluctance to eat or drink and indifference to everything going on around them; severe depressions with psychotic symptoms, or if the depression constitutes a life-threatening condition, ECT is the treatment of choice. ECT may also be suitable if the person has responded well to such treatment previously. Severe depressions in pregnant women and new mothers can be treated with ECT. Relief of symptoms is noticeable after just a few treatments (See Chapter 18).

When is light treatment recommended?

In seasonal affective disorder (SAD), especially the variant known as winter blues, light treatment is the primary recommendation (see also Chapters 3 and 18).

When are psychological treatments recommended?

Mild and certain moderate depressions can be treated with psychological treatment methods alone (see also Chapter 19). People, who want to understand their own depressive symptoms on the basis of their life history, are suitable subjects for psychological forms of treatment.

A person who succumbs to a mild depression for the first time should preferably be treated with psychological methods. Depression provoked by a trying situation, such as unemployment, divorce, relationship problems, or isolation, is usually relieved by means of psychological therapies and psychosocial measures.

Depressed children and young people should also be treated primarily with psychological methods, even for severe depression. They very often need to strengthen their self-confidence, and they can achieve this by means of various psychological treatments with elements of educational methodology, in which they learn to handle situations in life that may lead to depression. The therapist may serve as a model if children or young people lack functioning relationships with their parents. Sometimes therapy with the whole family is important.

When is combination treatment recommended?

When symptoms are acute, combining antidepressant treatment with psychotherapy is advisable. Antidepressants stabilize mood and reduce impulsiveness, while psychological treatments provide opportunities for a person to gain insight and find new survival strategies.

With antidepressants, certain people experience prompt relief from their symptoms, but cannot cope with their lives and relapse into old reaction patterns. These people should be given the chance to attend psychological treatment, so as to learn how to avoid new depressions by, for example, not taking on too much work, subjecting themselves to stress or choosing the wrong partner.

The therapist is an important discussion partner in reviewing the conflicts that have caused the depression. When a person's anguish has decreased, their mood has normalized and reality is no longer perceived as entirely black, their new way of experiencing reality allows them to consider their perception of the world when they were depressed.

Combination treatment with antidepressants and psychotherapy is often used for depressed people with personality disturbances. It should always be chosen for people suffering from persistent depression (dysthymia), and in treating people who suffer from depression with anguish.

The combination of lithium medication with psychological forms of treatment has a favourable effect on people with manic-depressive illness. The psychological treatment helps them to understand the course of the illness, and also lessens the psychological consequences in the event of relapse. The primary feature of combination treatment is that, besides the relief from depressive symptoms attained with antidepressants, people learn to deal with their stress and susceptibility towards anguish and depression.

When is social rehabilitation recommended?

Social rehabilitation combined with supportive therapy is aimed at training the depressed individual, increasing their capacity to cope with everyday life or work assignments. This form of training includes learning to get on with others. Social rehabilitation measures are usually combined with medication in the care of schizophrenics and alcohol or drugs abusers who simultaneously suffer from depression. Social rehabilitation is also necessary for depressed people whose work capacity is sharply reduced.

How is depression treated when it results from another illness?

If depression develops in conjunction with another illness, the latter should always be treated first. The same also applies to any abuse of alcohol, illicit drugs, and the like. An attempt should also be made to eliminate stress and conflict, which may be a precipitating or aggravating factor in depression.

How can a depression relapse be prevented?

Preventing relapse of a depressive illness is very important. Most people who have been depressed more than once usually recognize the symptoms of relapse. These may initially be only of a psychological nature; for example, feeling sensitive and turning down invitations from friends. In due course more severe symptoms develop, in the form of insomnia, lack of energy, anguish, worry, and despondency.

After completion of a course of antidepressant or psychological treatment, attention should be paid to whether the person continues to feel well or whether symptoms recur. Depression is commonly treated for 6 months at the maximum dose tried out during the first weeks of treatment. After 6 months, the dosage is usually reduced. However, if signs of deterioration are detected and the depression is visibly returning, the treatment dosage should be raised. This procedure should be repeated until the depressed person feels well. The same pattern should apply for psychological treatments.

16

Treatment with antidepressant medication

➲ Key points

- Symptoms and severity of depression are extremely variable; therefore it is important to tailor antidepressant treatment to the individual person.

- Tricyclic and tetracyclic antidepressants (TCAs) have very good effects in treatment of severely depressed people, melancholics, and those with compulsive disorders, but have many side effects.

- Selective serotonin reuptake inhibitors (SSRIs), Serotonin and noradrenaline reuptake inhibitors (SNRIs) and other new antidepressants, lack many of the side-effects of TCAs. They are suitable for long-term treatment of depression, compulsive disorders, panic attacks, and premenstrual syndromes.

- Melatonergic antidepressants have a beneficial effect on sleep and are used in treatment of depressions and anxiety disorders.

- Most antidepressant medication offers relief within 4–6 weeks.

- Lithium is the most effective and thoroughly tested agent for the treatment of manic-depressive illness.

Antidepressants are first choice to treat severe, and some types of moderate, depression. There are a variety of medications available with different mechanisms of action, use, and side effects.

Types of antidepressants

The symptoms and severity of depression are extremely variable from one individual to another. It is therefore important to tailor the treatment: choosing an antidepressant drug with an effect and side effect profile that suits the individual person. Routine prescription of antidepressants is wrong. To choose the right drug, doctors must: study in detail the person's clinical symptoms; take into account previous history of illness; and note any treatment they have received previously. Antidepressant medication is also used to treat anxiety, premenstrual dysphoric disorder, and pain.

Non-selective monoamine reuptake inhibitors

Tricyclic and tetracyclic antidepressants (TCAs)

TCAs are also sometimes called the 'older antidepressants' as they have been used in treating depressions since 1950. These drugs also have good and well-documented effects in long-term and preventive treatment of depression. TCAs benefit severely depressed people, and good results are attained from using them to treat melancholia and compulsive disorders.

Side effects of tricyclic antidepressants

TCAs cause a whole range of side effects. They reduce digestive activity, and can cause palpitations, dry mouth, constipation, and urinary retention. It is therefore important for people being treated with TCAs to have an adequate intake of bulk and fibre-rich foods. Dry membranes, especially in the eyes, may be a problem. Mouth dryness may also cause dental cavities. Reduced libido is not uncommon. Weight gain, fatigue, sleep problems, dizziness and low blood pressure, and reduced attentiveness can also occur. Elderly people may sometimes become confused.

Selective serotonin reuptake inhibitors (SSRIs)

SSRIs have a specific capacity to increase the concentration of serotonin in the central nervous system and were launched in the USA at the end of 1987. SSRIs are among the most widely prescribed antidepressants worldwide. It is no exaggeration to state that they have revolutionized the treatment of depression and have fewer side effects than TCAs. The risk of a deliberate overdose being lethal is small.

The fact that they have fewer side effects on the heart and the digestive system make SSRIs suitable for long-term preventive treatment of depression, and also in care of the elderly. Another advantage of the SSRIs is their effectiveness against compulsive disorders, panic attacks, and premenstrual syndromes.

Side effects of SSRIs

SSRIs lack many side-effects of TCAs. Side effects are as a rule temporary, but frequent and regular contact with the doctor is necessary. The main reason why frequent visits to the doctor are desirable is that the effects of SSRIs do not become apparent until after 2-4 weeks from the start of treatment, and the depressed person needs support to understand the course of the illness and the treatment. Sexual dysfunction, insomnia, nausea, diarrhoea, headache, and weight loss are among the principal side effects. It has also been reported that SSRIs may induce restlessness, disquiet, brooding, and suicidal thoughts in adolescents and young people.

Serotonin and noradrenaline reuptake inhibitors (SNRIs)

SNRI's lack many of the side effects of TCAs and are used to treat major depression, especially in cases that fail to respond to selective serotonin reuptake inhibitors (SSRIs). SNRIs influence levels in the central nervous system of both serotonin and noradrenaline.

Side effects of SNRIs

At low doses nausea, sexual disturbances, and insomnia may occur. At higher doses, increased blood pressure has been observed.

Monoamine oxidase (MAO) inhibitors and reversible inhibitors of MAO-A (RIMAs)

MAO inhibitors are a long standing group of antidepressants. There are two types of MAO inhibitor: the classic, non-reversible type, which is not usually used, and the reversible type, also known as RIMA.

Side effects of MAO and RIMAs

The side effects that occur are dizziness, nausea, and insomnia. RIMAs are used to treat major depression, atypical and refractory depression, as well as social phobias and panic attacks.

Melatonergic antidepressants

These antidepressants give relatively early symptom relief in depression and have beneficial effects on sleep, but do not cause sedation during the day time. They have also been successfully used alongside lithium in bipolar disorder and in the therapy of seasonal depression. They have few gastrointestinal side effects and do not affect sexual function, but may cause nausea and dizziness. This is important when treating males who often avoid antidepressants because of sexual side effects. Liver function tests are recommended in conjunction with this treatment.

Anticonvulsants

Anticonvulsant agents have been tried in major depression with good effect.

Combination of pharmacological treatments

In people who do not respond to treatment with a single antidepressant, especially after other medication has previously been tried, combining antide-pressants is recommended.

How long should treatment last?

As a rule, depressive symptoms are alleviated within 4–6 weeks of antidepres-sant treatment starting. To prevent a relapse, the treatment continues for at least 6 months longer, preferably 12 months. This is known as 'maintenance treatment'. Only after this period is there any certainty that recovery from the depressive episode has taken place. The antidepressant dosage should then be progressively reduced over a period of 2–4 weeks and, if the depressive symptoms are entirely gone, can be discontinued entirely. If the depressive symptoms recur, the person should once more be prescribed antidepressants at the same high dosage as during the previous 6 month period.

Side effects in general

Approximately, one-fifth of all people who receive antidepressant medication are troubled by side effects. These are often temporary. After a few weeks, most people have become accustomed to their medication. One way of mini-mizing the risk of side effects is by gradually raising the dosage. New antide-pressants have much milder side effects than their predecessors. Many people take these new drugs without any adverse effect whatsoever, while others incur side effects as early as the second day of treatment.

Addictiveness

Another issue is whether antidepressants are habit-forming or addictive. TCAs have been used long enough, and by enough people, to say that they are non-addictive. Nor are there any reports indicating that the newer antidepressants are addictive.

Risk of precipitating suicidal behaviour

People treated with antidepressants should be carefully supported by doctors and family, especially people with a history of previous suicide attempts and ongoing suicidal thoughts. The increase in suicide risk during treatment with antidepressants is due to the fact that the physical symptoms and energy improve quicker than emotions and the person continues, during the first weeks of the treatment, to find life hopeless and pointless.

Some antidepressants may even exacerbate the person's anxiety and in some people increases suicidality during the first few weeks of treatment. This applies particularly to people who suffer from depression with anxiety. Anxiety reducing drugs and sedative medication can be used to alleviate those symptoms. Every depressed person must be monitored thoroughly by means of frequent medical consultations until improvement takes place.

Combining alcohol and drugs with antidepressants

Some depressed people use alcohol or narcotics to relieve their anxiety. Self-treatment of this kind results in undesired side effects. Brain function, which is already disturbed by depression, is negatively affected by alcohol or drug consumption. Sleep is disturbed. Anyone taking antidepressant drugs should therefore avoid drinking alcohol and abstain completely from taking narcotics. Successful treatment with antidepressants has proved not only to relieve depression but also reduces people's craving for alcohol and drugs.

Antidepressants during pregnancy and breastfeeding

Caution should be exercised in prescribing antidepressants for pregnant women. These drugs pass through the placenta and are transferred to the fetus in small quantities, with a risk of the fetus being affected. Women who succumb to depression after childbirth can be treated with antidepressant medication if they are not breastfeeding.

In mild and moderate depression, psychological forms of treatment are a choice for pregnant and lactating women. Lithium and tranquillizers are not recommended during pregnancy and breastfeeding. If the mother's condition requires lithium treatment, she should refrain from breastfeeding. In severe depression an electroconvulsive treatment (ECT) can be used (see chapter 18).

Treatment of manic-depressive illness

The most effective and thoroughly tested agent for the treatment of manic-depressive illness and mania is lithium, which is deemed to be the medicine that best stabilizes mood. Lithium is used both to cure manic-depressive states and to prevent relapse into mania and depression.

With lithium treatment, people may incur such symptoms as nausea, diarrhoea and vomiting, tremors, and coordination difficulties. People treated with lithium are often thirsty, and it is important for this thirst to be quenched with water and not high-calorie drinks, to prevent weight gain. Coffee or tea in large quantities (more than ten cups a day) can increase urinary excretion of lithium, thus reducing its therapeutic effect.

It is important to start lithium treatment as soon as the diagnosis of manic-depressive illness or mania is verified, in order to counteract relapse and prevent the course from becoming chronic. The more promptly treatment is commenced, the better the results. Lithium treatment involves no risk of addiction and helps to reduce suicidality.

17

Sexuality, depression, and antidepressant medication

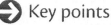 Key points

- Sexual problems most frequently experienced in depression are: reduced sexual desire and arousal, failure to achieve orgasm, and ejaculation problems.

- Psychological factors are very important in sexual relations and depressed people often feel a lack of interest in relationships.

- Depressed people who abuse alcohol have more severe sexual disturbances.

- Depressed people should definitely not refrain from sexual activity, even if full intercourse is not feasible. Tenderness and sensual experiences may also provide pleasure.

Sexual activity and desire may alter when suffering from depression. Some antidepressant medications can also affect sexuality, but when depression is cure sexual problems usually cease to be a problem.

Sexuality in depression

Sexual problems in depression are often described as reduced sexual desire and arousal, and failure to achieve orgasm or ejaculation. Just over a third of depressed men suffer from premature ejaculation. Almost half complain of delayed ejaculation. Approximately 30% of depressed women complain of reduced sexual desire or absence of orgasm. As sexuality is the most intimate part of our lives, it may be difficult for people to raise the subject of sexual problems spontaneously during a medical consultation.

In investigating sexual problems experienced by depressed people, it is important to compare their current condition with that before they fell ill. The most frequent problem is reduced interest in sex. Psychological factors are very important in sexual relations. A depressed person often feels powerless to act, with a lack of interest in relationships.

Depressed people who abuse alcohol have more severe sexual disturbances than those who do not, as alcohol abuse can diminish sexual activity. Cannabis and cocaine may boost sexual desire in the short term, but in severe abuse an inhibitory effect on sexuality has been demonstrated.

Antidepressants and sexuality

Sometimes it is difficult to determine whether a person's unsatisfactory sexual relations are due to depression or to their antidepressant medication. Some antidepressant drugs disturb human sexual functioning. Reduced libido (sexual desire), erection difficulties, and absence of ejaculation and orgasm are side effects of medication, which cease as soon as one recovers from depression. Lithium and melatonergic antidepressants are free of sexual side effects.

If a depressed person's sexual disturbances are troublesome and sexual life is essential to the person concerned, the doctor may prescribe an antidepressant that does not disturb sexual functioning. However, the essential consideration is for the depressed person to become free from depression as rapidly as possible. As soon as the depression has been remedied, sexual functioning also recovers. It is therefore sometimes worth accepting side effects perceived as troublesome at the beginning of treatment if the medication is considered the most suitable.

Assisting libido

Regarding long-term maintenance treatment of depression, the person should ask the doctor to choose medicines that are known for not causing sexual side effects. The doctor may also prescribe a break of 1 or 2 days in the course of antidepressants before a planned sexual activity—a 'drug holiday', as it is called.

Depressed people should definitely not refrain from sexual activity, even if full intercourse is not feasible. In mild or moderate depression in particular, it is very often the mental inhibition and incapacity to act that impedes performance of the sexual act. To arouse desire, sexual foreplay is important even if it does not necessarily always culminate in full intercourse. Tenderness and sensual experiences may also provide as much satisfaction as the sexual act itself. Mental and physical closeness is important and should also be tended during a period of depression.

Sometimes people may become fixated on their unsatisfactory sex lives even after the depression has passed and their sexual functioning, as such, is in fact normal. Psychological treatment methods usually help to remedy this kind of deadlock. In some cases, counselling may be important to discuss the practicalities of sexual technique.

18

Electroconvulsive therapy and light therapy

 Key points

Two forms of treatment for depression that can be used alongside or instead of antidepressant medication are: electroconvulsive therapy and light therapy.

Electroconvulsive therapy (ECT) is a tried and tested, effective treatment for severe depression of a melancholic nature with marked psychomotor inhibition that is unresponsive to antidepressant medication. ECT has very rapid effects.

- For pregnant women or new mothers suffering from severe depression, ECT is an option when psychological treatment has not helped.

- ECT causes no brain damage and roughly 80% of severely depressed people show improvement.

- Transcranial magnetic stimulation is a milder treatment than ECT, particularly used for treating seasonal depression.

- Light therapy has proved to be a good method of treating recurrent seasonal depression or SAD (seasonal affective mood disorder), especially winter depressions.

Electroconvulsive therapy

ECT is a tried and tested, effective treatment for severe depression that is unresponsive to antidepressant medication. These people wish neither to eat nor drink. They do not react to thirst, and there is a risk of the illness culminating in death from dehydration. Such people also have reduced reactions to pain stimuli, and their failure to perceive pain increases a risk of self-injury. Melancholic people who have severe delusions concerning punishment and guilt, notions that they suffer from some serious and incurable illness, or intense feelings of panic are also suitable candidates for ECT. ECT may also be used in the care of depressed people who are strikingly remote from reality and who show clear psychotic symptoms, with delusions and hallucinations.

For pregnant women or new mothers suffering from severe depression, ECT may be an option when psychological treatment in the acute phase has not helped. In severe manic states that do not respond to medication, ECT is also usually effective.

ECT has very rapid effects: alleviation of depressive symptoms takes place after only a few sessions. Unfortunately, ECT has fallen into disrepute. The main reason for this is that the method was very often used in the past in an unselective manner.

Effect mechanism

In ECT, stimulation of the brain takes place with a minimal quantity of electrical energy. This stimulation provokes a brief epileptic attack. ECT does not cause brain damage, and approximately 80% of people treated show improvement. After a single treatment session, many people experience short-lived relief. In most cases, the depression relieving effect is felt already after three to four sessions. This improvement applies to most depressive symptoms. Physical symptoms, such as sleep and appetite, are relieved and psychomotor inhibition also decreases. Mental symptoms, such as anxiety and apathy, are also alleviated and mood is normalized.

Procedure

Between 5 and 12 ECT sessions are usually given, at a rate of 3 a week. On average, a person is treated between six and eight times. If the first series of ECT sessions do not work, another series may be given after 2 months.

The treatment is administered under anaesthetic and the whole procedure, including preparations, anaesthesia, and awakening, lasts roughly half an hour. The actual epileptic attack lasts for 20–60 seconds. After a series of sessions is completed, maintenance treatment with antidepressant drugs and psychological forms of treatment is given.

Side-effects of ECT

Certain people may suffer temporary memory disturbances after treatment, owing to the brief reduction in oxygen to the brain. People may have a memory gap covering the period of treatment, or have difficulty in remembering what happened immediately before, during, and after the session. Ordinary headache occurs in roughly 30% of people given ECT. Transitory muscular aches and nausea are less common. Sometimes the person suffers tooth fractures from the muscle cramps.

📄 Robert, aged 41

Robert is 41 years old and has a wife, Helen. A year ago, their son Andrew died in a road accident. Two of his friends who were in the car with him survived. The driver was severely injured and is still in hospital. The accident took place on the day after Andrew left secondary school.

Andrew and his friends had wanted to go and celebrate the fact that one friend had a job at a summer camp. Robert had quarrelled with Andrew just before they left, as Andrew's whole last month before leaving school had been one big series of celebrations. For various reasons, their relationship was tense. Robert knew that Andrew smoked hash and perhaps also used other drugs. He also sniffed glue. This period of abuse came to an end when, after being caught committing a minor crime, he was treated by the youth psychiatric team in his local area. Helen always hoped that Andrew would grow out of it. There were many quarrels and even physical fights, between the father and son. She was always trying to smooth things over.

After the police announced his son's death, Robert became apathetic and did not react to what was going on around him. The symptoms persisted. He began sinking into himself, and neglected his work, the house, and the garden, where he usually enjoyed pottering about. In short, slow sentences, Robert sometimes stated that God had punished him as he himself was the cause of Andrew's death. He also reproached himself for ruining his wife's life, and for the shame that Robert had brought upon the family.

Robert lost his desire to live. On one occasion he carefully polished his gun, sat, and stared ahead. He refused to take antidepressants so his doctor ensured that Robert was admitted to a psychiatric hospital. ECT was prescribed, and Robert underwent marked improvement after six sessions. Robert has now gone back to work and feels fairly well, but although everything has returned to normal he does not believe that his life will ever be the same again.

Transcranial magnetic stimulation

Transcranial magnetic stimulation (TMS) is a milder treatment than ECT. Electromagnetic stimulation of the left frontal lobe of the brain can alleviate depression. This takes place without causing cramp, nor is there any need for the person to be anaesthetized. Properly conducted treatment is considered to be free of complications and side effects. It is hoped that in the future, TMS can replace ECT, however, more research is needed.

Vagus nerve stimulation

Another treatment that is being tested is weak electric stimulation of the vagus nerve. This is the longest nerve in the body, running from the brain stem to the base of the spine as well as to several organs and the heart. When the vagus nerve activates it triggers a relaxation response. Enhanced mood has been reported among a group of chronically depressed people that have responded poorly to other treatment. These results demand continuous evaluation, and definitive clinical trials are awaited; therefore, this treatment is still considered as experimental.

Deep brain stimulation

Deep brain stimulation (inserting electrodes into the brain) is used in Parkinson's disease, and is effective in reducing tremors associated with this disease. The technique can also be used to treat severe obsessive-compulsive disorders.

Light therapy

Light therapy has proved to be effective in treating recurrent seasonal depression or SAD (seasonal affective mood disorder). People with winter depression, a particular form of SAD, respond well to light treatment. Predominantly women aged 20–50 suffer from winter fatigue and winter depression. Typical symptoms are fatigue despite sleep, and a reduction in physical activity combined with increased appetite, leading to weight gain.

Effect mechanisms and effectiveness

The effect mechanisms of light therapy have not been fully established, but it is known to influence the biological daily rhythm of the body. Light entering the retina regulates our biological clock by reducing secretion of the hormone melatonin in the blood. Melatonin serves as a rhythmic regulator of sleep and wakefulness. Receptors in the skin also react to the rhythm of light and darkness.

Light therapy has positive effects on winter depressions. Results are usually noticeable after only a few treatment sessions. As many as 80% of people are entirely relieved of their symptoms: physical and mental energy increases and mood improves after only ten light therapy sessions.

On the other hand, light therapy does not have the same positive therapeutic effects on people with non-seasonal depression and in people with SAD who suffer from personality disorders. Nor may favourable results be expected from light therapy if a person suffering from winter depression also simultaneously has another form of depression. In these cases, treatment must be combined with some other form of care, or an entirely different type of treatment must be chosen.

Procedure

Light therapy is initiated with a light box that directs bright light downwards to the person. Sessions start with brief exposure to this bright light, and the duration of exposure is gradually increased. Both the strength of the bright light, and the duration of sessions can vary. Short sessions are compensated for with a brighter light.

To maximize the effect all surfaces in the room, including the doors, are painted white. The floor is very light, with no pattern. The windows are also covered with curtains so that no daylight enters. The person is dressed in white and must keep their eyes open as the light works through the retina, which is connected to the brain. The light is never directed *straight* at the eyes. Overhead strip lighting casts *indirect* light, irrespective of one's position in the room.

Light therapy is usually given in a series of ten sessions and may be adapted to the individual's needs. The person can continue with light-therapy sessions at home two or three times a week throughout the winter period, with special lamps.

Side effects

There are side effects for light therapy. Some people may incur headaches, especially those who suffer from migraine. Eye irritation may also occur. Some people, or those who suffer from manic-depressive illness may become elated (hypomanic), or mania may be triggered.

19

Psychological forms of treatment

➡ Key points

◆ Psychological support is helpful for depressed people, alongside antidepressant or other biological treatment.

◆ Antidepressive medication gives depressed people physical energy to undertake therapy.

◆ Psychological therapies as the sole treatment of depression are recommended for: pregnant and lactating women, people with relationship problems, or when unemployment, economic problems, and other crisis situations cause depression.

◆ Cognitive therapy (CT) and cognitive behavioural therapy (CBT) clarify depressed people's views of reality affected by negative perceptions of themselves and the world.

◆ Interpersonal Psychotherapy (IPT) focuses on communicating with other people.

◆ In counselling, the depressed person is given an opportunity to explore their life by addressing and resolving specific problems.

◆ A trusting, stable, and secure relationship between the depressed person and their therapist is vital.

Psychological treatment has been found helpful in the treatment of depression. Several surveys have shown that cognitive behavioural therapy and interpersonal therapy are highly effective in remedying mild and moderate depression. Scientific studies indicate that 85% of people receiving combination treatment with antidepressant drugs and psychological therapy are cured of their depression.

You cannot stop the birds of sorrow
and distress flying over your head.
But you can prevent them
from nesting in your hair.

Chinese proverb

Psychological therapies as treatment methods

The view that depressed people should be treated with *either* antidepressant medication *or* psychological methods has been abandoned by modern psychiatrists. All depressed people, regardless of whether they are treated with antidepressants (see Chapter 16) or other biological treatment methods (Chapter 18) can benefit from psychological support.

With medication, a depressed person's mood improves relatively rapidly. On the other hand, their view of themselves and others often lags behind. Psychological treatment methods are therefore recommended to enable depressed people to find appropriate strategies for coping with their problems in life. It is important for those concerned to learn to recognize emotions that were previously suppressed, and give vent to their sadness instead of bottling it up. Through psychotherapy, people learn to understand and integrate life events and experiences. Antidepressant medication can give depressed people the physical energy required to learn, through psychotherapy, to become more observant and aware of how they react to stressful life situations.

When psychological treatment is recommended

Psychological therapies as the sole form of treatment are recommended for mild or moderate types of depression in:

◆ Pregnant and lactating women

◆ People with relationship and lifestyle problems such as divorce or unemployment

♦ Refugees with mild or moderate depression

♦ People of personality types with tendencies towards depression (see Chapter 13)

♦ People who find antidepressants unacceptable owing to their side effects

♦ People reluctant to take antidepressant medication

♦ People who have failed to respond to antidepressants treatment alone.

The effectiveness of psychological treatment depends on the person and the therapist forming a good working partnership. Stereotyped assumptions about which types of people are most likely to benefit from psychotherapy should be avoided: it is not only middle-class or well-educated people, females, or those under the age of 50 who can benefit. Nor should a person's social class, ethnic group, age, and sex determine their access to treatment.

What does psychological treatment involve?

Psychological treatment is a form of systematic 'talking cure' (psychotherapy) with well-defined objectives, provided by an authorized therapist. Psychotherapy exists in various forms. To date, the best evidence that depressive disorders may be treated effectively with psychotherapy relates to cognitive, cognitive behavioural, and interpersonal therapy. The choice of form of psychotherapy is made partly with reference to the depressed person's problems, symptoms, personality, and ways of functioning and relating to others. Personal preference should be taken into account. During the first 2-3 sessions, the therapist makes an assessment and shares it with the person, who then agrees on which type of psychological treatment is most suitable.

One purpose of psychological treatment is to mobilize a person's energy and strengthen their self-confidence, thus enabling them to take control of their own lives. In the course of treatment, people gain new experience and reinterpret the old. In due course, depressed people gain a better understanding of the reasons for their depression and make better use of their own resources through enhanced self-knowledge.

Types of psychological therapies in depression

The various forms of psychological therapy differ regarding method and the therapist–patient relationship. In some forms the therapist is active, questioning, guiding, and encouraging, while in others they are more neutral and let the patient lead.

Cognitive therapy (CT) and cognitive behavioural therapy (CBT)

The objective of CT and CBT is to reduce depressive symptoms by finding alternative ways for people to see themselves, others, and the world in general. Through therapy, they learn to redefine their frames of reference and change their ways of interpreting their perceptions of threatening and stressful situations that usually trigger feelings of hurt, anxiety, and hopelessness—feelings that, in turn, may result in depression. People also learn to reassess their previous strategies in order to cope with stressful situations by developing new ways of dealing with them.

The goal of the therapy is to change negative thinking patterns, replacing them with a more realistic self-image, and empowering people to influence their own situation. One important part of the treatment is to learn stress management. Negative thoughts and perceptions usually arise when performing a task or solving a problem. Instead of trying different strategies for performing the task, depressed people feel that they have failed if the one and only strategy they try proves inadequate.

CT and CBT are also used to treat anxiety problems, personality disorders, substance abuse, and eating disorders. There are specific guidelines for both CT and CBT, covering the content of each session, and the homework assignments that are prescribed.

In both CT and CBT, the therapist is active. They pose questions, guide the person, and impart structure to every session. During the sessions, specific situations in which the depressed person experiences problems are systematically raised and discussed. In the course of this process, the person's thoughts and views are explored. Such thoughts as 'I'm a useless person', 'I'm no good at anything', 'I don't dare', 'I'm bound to fail', 'I never succeed', 'Everything's going wrong', and 'I'll get the sack' are analysed and described. Thoughts of this type are associated with a fundamentally negative view and interpretation of oneself and others. In the course of the therapy, the therapist and person attempt to examine alternative approaches and replace the negative thoughts by new, positive ones.

Both short-term and long-term treatment with CT and CBT are given. The short-term therapy comprises of 20 sessions and the longer 60. Each session lasts roughly an hour. The person usually attends sessions once or twice a week initially, and less frequently towards the end of the treatment.

Short-term treatment with CT and CBT is evidence based in the treatment of depressions. It takes longer to achieve lasting change in people with more problematic social and personality functioning or with chronic relapsing depression. The objective of the treatment is to improve depressed people's self-esteem by changing their opinions of themselves and others, and to teach them to form close relationships.

Behavioural therapy

This is a form of structured therapy in which problems are solved and symptoms relieved by modification of dysfunctional behaviour. BT is an option in the treatment of depressions characterized by severe anxiety and phobias. In this treatment, in the therapist's presence, depressed people are subjected to the stressful situations that trigger their anxiety, phobias, and depression. Not only behaviour, but also the events and situations that provoke it, are explored. Graded exposure to feared situations is one of the most common behavioural treatment methods and also has good effects in the treatment of phobias, panic attacks, and compulsive behaviour. Through progressive habituation to disagreeable situations, the person's symptoms are reduced or completely eliminated.

Dialectic behavioural therapy (DBT)

DBT is a long-term treatment in which people are taught skills for regulating and accepting their emotions. Their capacity for interpersonal effectiveness is also enhanced.

DBT is a form of therapy which has proved beneficial in treating women with personality disorders who make repeated suicide attempts. The treatment consists of individual therapy and group social-skills training and focuses on situations that provoke anxiety, depressive feelings, and suicidal behaviour. People also learn how, in new ways, which improves their social capacity to regulate strong moods such as anger, rage, aggressiveness, shame, hopelessness, and sorrow.

Treatment is usually scheduled for a year or longer. The therapist is active and encouraging. Encouragement is an important part of the treatment, as depressed and suicidal people have often lacked it previously in life. DBT can also be combined with antidepressant medication.

DBT sessions vary between 50 and 60 minutes in length once or twice a week and are adapted to the person's capacity. In group therapy, people meet for about 2 hours weekly over a year or more. At each group meeting, the skills that people have learnt in previous sessions are built upon. There is also scope for repeated skills training if the person has not attained the level that, in consultation with the therapist, is considered satisfactory.

Interpersonal psychotherapy (IPT)

IPT is a structured form of supportive therapy in which interpersonal events are linked to moods or other problems. In this therapy, systematic attention is paid to current personal relationship problems, incapacity to handle transitions, role conflicts, and losses. Particular emphasis is laid on the depressed person's way of communicating with other people. The person and therapist choose to focus on relationships: marriage, the family, with parents, in the workplace, or on new roles in life owing, for example, to divorce, a new job, or becoming a parent. Each problem area is analysed using specific techniques. The aim is to boost self-confidence by improving the social skills of the depressed person.

This form of psychotherapy is of limited duration. Treatment consists of about 20 sessions lasting 50–60 minutes. The IPT can also be given as a long-term form of treatment, and may last between 1 and 2 years with sessions once or twice a week. To prevent relapse, treatment lasting two or more years is recommended. There have been promising reports of this type of psychotherapy following postpartum depression.

Psychodynamic psychotherapy

The aim of the treatment is for people to gain an insight into their own life histories and the underlying conflicts that result in their anxiety and depression. Through the therapy, they replace their old, inappropriate ways of resolving conflicts with more realistic strategies. These insights give people better self-knowledge and self-esteem, and increased independence. The therapy is concluded with a phase-out of the depressed person's dependence on the therapist that has usually arisen in the course of the treatment, enabling the person to work through their own problems unaided.

Psychodynamic therapy is based on a range originating in different schools of psychoanalysis. Psychoanalysis was founded by Sigmund Freud, and his many followers' theories form the foundations of this type of therapy. People must be interested in exploring their emotional lives, past and present, and have the capacity for symbolic thinking and verbal expression of emotions.

One problem that depressed people often have difficulty with, is a conflict between feeling dependent on other people and, at the same time, having a strong wish to be independent. By placing current situations in perspective, people try during therapy to understand why, for example, they become dependent and form connections with men or women of a certain type; and why, invariably, these relationships break down and depression ensues. People learn to see how the pattern repeats itself and why they are failing to change.

In psychodynamic psychotherapy, the therapist is more of a neutral listener and less of an active adviser than in, cognitive psychotherapy or IPT. During therapy, people learn to change their attitude from one of preoccupation with their own symptoms, to readiness to examine their own problems by expressing their emotions and conflicts in words.

In psychodynamic psychotherapy, the therapist and person meet once or twice a week, usually for 2 years. To prevent relapse and a chronic course of depression, treatment lasting several years is sometimes recommended. This is similar to recommendations for long-term treatment with antidepressants to prevent relapse and chronic development. The sessions last 50 minutes and usually take place at the same time and on the same day every week. Shorter treatments, lasting from 3 months to a year, are also given. In this kind of short-term treatment with psychodynamic psychotherapy, the person and therapist usually decide in advance how long the treatment is to last and what it should focus on.

Counselling

Many depressed people, often men, are not interested in exploring their emotional lives; nor, perhaps, are they accustomed to describing them verbally. In these cases, people can receive counselling and/or supportive psychotherapy, where the depressed person is given an opportunity to explore and clarify ways of living that give a greater sense of well-being. Specific problems can be addressed and resolved. The depressed person is taught how to make decisions, cope with crises, improve relationships with others, and/or work through conflicts. Counsellors focus on 'here and now' choices. Most counsellors apply humanistic, process-experiential, and psychodynamic principles.

Supportive psychotherapy

This is very helpful in every course of antidepressant treatment. Many psychiatrists, and some General Practitioners, are trained to conduct supportive therapy. They can establish a rapport with the depressed person that is characterized by understanding, empathy, and an ability to tackle the depressed person's painful feelings and anxiety. Doctors can both inspire hope at the darkest times when the depression is at its worst and, using educational methods, show how depressed people and their families can deal with various stressful situations.

Family therapy and couple therapy

For certain mildly and moderately depressed people, couple or family therapy is recommended to resolve the relationship conflicts that have caused the depression. The communication pattern in families with a depressed member is often complex. This pattern needs to be sorted out, and the family members must learn to communicate with and understand one another. Therapy can clarify the roles assigned to the various members and the roles they would, in fact, like to play. The whole family is also taught to cope with various types of stress.

Group therapy

A form of therapy known as 'group (or gestalt) therapy', in which the depressed person can practise using various social skills and socializing with others, may also be used. Couple, family, and group forms of therapy are not used in the acute phase of depression. Instead, they may be successfully applied in the rehabilitation phase and to prevent relapse. All these forms of therapy can be combined with antidepressant medication.

Non-verbal forms of therapy

People who have difficulty in expressing themselves in words can use other techniques, such as art therapy, handicrafts, and music, to get in touch with their feelings and experiences. By concentrating on non-verbal perceptions that relate to their senses, depressed people can come into contact with their feelings. In this way, an insight may be afforded into depressed people's development and various events during their upbringing that are connected with the way they perceive the present-day situation and their current depression.

Physical forms of therapy, such as physiotherapy or massage, may also help many people. Yoga and meditation are widely used as means of obtaining new strength. This tranquillity and reduction in stress may, in many cases, prevent depression and relapse.

Changing one's doctor or psychotherapist

Sometimes, in the course of treatment, people may get frustrated with, or even begin to dislike, the therapist or doctor that they initially regarded as very good. During treatment, a 'therapeutic process' develops both consciously and unconsciously, and the same types of feeling develop towards the therapist that the person usually has towards others, such as parents, siblings, teachers, classmates, partners, colleagues, and friends. Understanding these feelings and reaction patterns is an important part of the therapeutic process and should be communicated. If negative feelings towards the care giver persist, in spite of elucidating them, one should discuss changing to another care giver.

Combination of psychological treatment with antidepressants

All psychological treatment can be combined with antidepressants and vice versa. For many depressed people, the combination of biological and psychological forms of treatment is very beneficial.

20

Advice to family members

⮕ Key points

- Relatives can give support by ensuring the depressed person receives professional help and by offering assistance during the course of the illness.

- Psychological and moral support where one listens, inspires, and counteracts isolation through body language and words is very important.

- Depressed people are often 'hungry for love' and highly sensitive to lack of appreciation. It is important to confirm that they are liked and needed.

- Relatives should, with confidence, express the hope that the depressed person will feel better soon, although recovery may be slow, with setbacks.

- Those suffering from a mild or moderate depression should be helped and encouraged to go to work. Activity counteracts passivity and flight from ordinary life.

Providing help and support for a depressed person can be a mentally arduous and difficult task. In purely practical terms, it may mean being the only one looking after the home, children, and finances, as the depressed partner cannot manage these tasks. Seek a support for yourself as living with and supporting a depressed person is emotionally and mentally draining. Relatives and friends must feel strong in themselves before they offer help. Having relatives and friends who care and support is one of the most important factors promoting health.

The words of grief kill none.
Dumb silence is what kills.
Speaking, we live.
Speechless, we die.
Listen, then, to my voice—a paltry flame that lights up the walls
of our cave.
There is no one here, there is nothing to fear as long as the word
exists and the flame is lit.

Translated from Olof Lagercrantz,
Swedish writer and poet (1911–2002)

When a family member is suffering from depression

Many depressed people say of themselves 'I don't recognize myself anymore.' Family members, too, may have the same feeling about depressed people: that their behaviour is not really recognizable. The irritation and impatience they may show others are, perhaps, entirely alien to their usual character. Sleep disturbances, lack of appetite, and anguish may be other early signs of depression. As the onset of depression is often not obvious and it takes time for all the symptoms to develop to the full, a relative may become used to the successive change in a person's behaviour and fail to seek professional help in time.

The despondent person's depressive ideas or deeply pessimistic view of life may 'infect' family members, who may succumb to a sense of despair and hopelessness. They may start uncritically believing what the depressed person says, thus unconsciously adopting the same attitude towards the outside world. As a relative one can give support by, first, ensuring that the depressed person receives professional help and, secondly, offering psychological and practical assistance during the course of the illness.

Professional help

Depressed people should always be encouraged to seek help. They are sometimes reluctant to go to the doctor or the psychologist, and a great deal of diplomacy may be required. A despondent person should not be rushed. It is important to try and understand what the resistance is about: it may be a sense of shame about being ill, or a distrust of medication. Many people are afraid of antidepressants and their side effects. Today, there are new antidepressants that have fairly few troublesome side effects. Certain types of depression can, moreover, be remedied with psychological methods or light treatment. If a depressed person shows strong resistance to seeking professional help, it may be helpful for a family member to ask a doctor for advice on how to proceed.

If a visit to the doctor has been booked, one should ask the depressed person for permission for someone to accompany him or her. A relative or friend can give the doctor valuable information about the despondent person's way of functioning socially, so that the doctor can assess which form of care is most appropriate. Relatives can sometimes describe the illness better than the sufferers themselves. Close contact with doctors is always very important, but should take place with the approval of the depressed person in question. In very profound depressions or in the event of suicide risk, however, relatives should contact a doctor even if they have not received the sufferer's permission: this may be a life-saving measure.

Psychological support

Psychological (emotional) support may be given through an attempt to understand how depressed people feel. One should listen and try to inspire the depressed person to counteract their tendency towards isolation.

Active listening

Showing that one hears and understands what depressed people are trying to convey is important, and one should confirm this by means of body language and words. When depressed people are feeling worst, one should not question their message. Even if one's own view is different, one should not interrupt or disagree. Despondent people very often cannot cope with conversation and argument. Such discussions should wait until they feel better.

Sometimes a severely despondent person may be in need of long talks in which the same issues recur. The repetition may seem burdensome to others, but it is an important part of a depressed person's way of working through their illness. Telephoning is helpful: a call may enhance the sufferer's mood, raising hopes of recovery. One should avoid telling depressed people that they should try to pull themselves together. This is ineffective, as severely despondent people are quite simply incapable of doing so. Over-optimistic encouragement is perceived as stressful.

Understanding

A relative's task is to try to comprehend how the depressed person feels. One should also convey sympathy and show an understanding that it may feel wearisome and arduous to be depressed. This kind of attitude may result in an outpouring of sorrow, which usually affords relief to despondent people. One should not interrupt a fit of crying by attempting to give consolation. Crying may be a healthy step towards healing.

Depressed people are highly sensitive to lack of appreciation and love. For them, it is important to obtain confirmation that they are liked and needed. Relatives who feel tired or irritated themselves, or think they have difficulty in showing the depressed person positive feelings, should ask someone else to look after them. Helpers must make sure that they themselves can relax and recover their strength. Even if they do not express their irritation, discontent, or lack of love verbally, their body language will reveal it to the depressed person, whose condition may deteriorate as a result.

Talk in a hope-inspiring way

Expressing understanding of the ordeal the depressed person is going through and showing empathy and compassion are important supportive measures. Relatives can share their own experience of setbacks, crises, and any periods of despondency they have had. This can help depressed people to realize that others understand what they are going through. Tell the depressed person that both medical and psychological treatment methods are available, and encourage them to seek help.

If a depressed person complains of troublesome side effects from antidepressants, they can be consoled with the advice that these usually pass, and encouraged to continue with the prescribed treatment. It usually takes time for the effects of medication or psychotherapy to become evident. In treatment with antidepressants, it takes 4–6 weeks before symptoms of depression begin to be alleviated; with psychotherapy, it takes longer.

When depressed people have recovered, family members should attempt to raise the issue of how to deal with any relapse that may occur. These relapses may occur frequently, or they may be several years apart. It is important to be prepared for the possibility of depression returning, and ensure that treatment is sought as promptly as possible.

Counteracting loneliness

One should stay in touch with those who are depressed, even if they declare it to be unnecessary. It is never right to leave a depressed person alone. Severely despondent people wish most of all to isolate themselves and not mix with anyone. However, solitude makes their condition worse.

Practical support

Nobody is useless in this world who lightens the burdens of another.
Charles Dickens, English author (1812–70)

Very often, depressed people have difficulty in collecting their thoughts. They also miss the overall picture, and see only parts of reality. Through practical assistance, despondent people can be prevented from losing their perspective. Above all, they should be helped to complete the course of treatment prescribed.

Depressed people often need practical help with continuous chores and duties. They can, for example, be accompanied to the doctor and assisted in carrying out errands, paying bills, and shopping, depending on how much they can manage unaided. If they are evidently beginning to regain their strength and capacity for action, they should be encouraged to perform their duties themselves. However, it is always enjoyable to do things with others even if one feels well, and it is therefore always a good idea to develop such habits in the family.

Support may also be given by a review and restructuring of workload. At times, specific measures are needed to go through all the depressed person's duties and ration the commitments. Sometimes a great deal of support is required to induce depressed people to stop reproaching themselves and feeling guilty about what they feel should be done, but they cannot cope with.

Financial transactions should be avoided, as those undertaken during depression are often ill advised and governed by exaggerated pessimism. Travel, too should be avoided as it does not usually provide any stimulation for a depressed person. One should not quarrel with a depressed person or bring up questions of separation or divorce, as this exacerbates depression and may contribute to suicidal thoughts. Seeking professional help to solve relationship problems instead of getting into constant conflicts is a practical option.

Seeking support for oneself

Living with and supporting a depressed person is emotionally and mentally draining; it is not easy to see the person's behaviour changing and emotional life becoming blunted. The pessimism and sense of hopelessness that characterizes depressed people may 'infect' others. When someone becomes depressed for the first time and there is no clear external cause triggering the depression, family members do not understand that it is an illness and, instead, perceive the depressed person as difficult, tiresome, tedious, or sluggish.

As depressed people often lack a sense of commitment, their partners often find themselves alone in dealing with practical tasks that were previously shared. It may be difficult to combine care of a depressed relative with one's own paid job, running the home, and looking after the children, who may be in the throes of an adolescent crisis, or with care of elderly parents who are physically ill. The helper may then start feeling anxious, helpless, or abandoned. In such a situation it is natural to be tired, and feelings of irritation, anxiety, and inadequacy are normal. Talking to someone may be beneficial. Sometimes talking to a friend is enough. However, if family members feel that they themselves are becoming despondent, they should obtain professional help.

Depressed people's children

Many children of depressed people have no one to talk to. Like adults, children need to talk about their situation, ask questions, and obtain answers about their parents' or other relatives' depression. Children also need to show their feelings and talk about their anxiety. It is paramount for them to know that their mother's or father's depression is not a child's fault. It is never wrong to talk to children about a family member's depression.

21

Self-help in depression

🔁 Key points

◆ It is particularly important not to overstrain oneself or stretch one's stress-tolerance limits if there is a tendency to become despondent.

◆ Telling others about how one feels and not bottling feelings up, makes problems seem smaller and more realistic.

◆ Encouraging a positive attitude towards life and stimulating tasks promote health and recovery from mental and physical illnesses.

◆ Focus on regular eating habits and a balanced diet with daily intake of fresh fruit and vegetables, rice, fish, and moderate quantities of bread, meat, and pasta. Slimming diets exacerbate depression and should be avoided.

◆ Physical activity distracts the mind from gloomy thoughts and diverts attention from disagreeable events that contribute to depression.

◆ Sleep problems are common in depression. Regular sleep habits are vital for revitalization of the central nervous system.

Food, exercise, light, routine, and relaxation are the aspects of life we ourselves can influence, and which can prevent certain types of depression. They can improve the results of medical or psychological treatment for depression, and hasten recovery.

Too weak for one more step,
too tired to raise your head,
bowed beneath the greyness of despair.
Be thankful, glad for the little things, the friendly, childish comforts.
The apple in your pocket, the storybook at home.
Little, little things, despised at times that radiate with life,
but gentle mainstays in the dead hours.

Translated from Karin Boye, Swedish poet (1900–41)

Every human being's life is governed by biological and psychological cycles, and regularity is important in diet and exercise, as well as sleep, work, and rest. Self-help involving adequate diet, exercise, sleep, stress management, and alcohol habits can both prevent depression from arising and, in the event, improve the results of treatment. The key to self-help is actively looking after one's body and mind. Many of us have, perhaps, grown up with bad habits in which we persist. It is essential to break these habits and become actively aware of oneself.

Stress management

It is particularly important not to overstrain oneself or stretch stress-tolerance limits if there is a tendency to become despondent. When one is despondent or depressed, a good start is to write a list of tasks waiting to be done, and then obtain a trusted person's help in trying to reassign priorities and eliminate commitments that are unnecessary or can be taken care of by someone else. This may sometimes help the guilt about all the tasks left undone. It is good to say no to new commitments and errands during a depressive period. When requested to take on a task, one should avoid promising anything on the spur of the moment.

Although it is important for a depressed person to slow down and take some time off work, it is nevertheless good to keep going to work when one is suffering from mild or moderate depression. People who are despondent or depressed would prefer to isolate themselves, which makes depression worse. For the recovery process, it is important not to lose touch with colleagues and friends. However, superiors should be informed and so a joint agreement can be reached on what must be done. In such situations, the option of being on part-time sick leave is a good one.

Relaxation, yoga, and meditation reduce tension and anxiety. Meditation is a relaxation method with ancient traditions from such oriental religions as Hinduism, Buddhism, Taoism, and Zen. The purpose of yoga and meditation is to enhance self-awareness while minimizing physiological and cerebral activity. Massage or a hot bath also have a relaxing effect.

Tending the mind

Telling others about how one feels and not bottling feelings up, makes problems seem smaller and more realistic. Depression often makes everything look black. One should therefore not make any important decisions while depressed.

Regular contact with at least one friend, relative, or someone else whom one can talk to should be striven for. It is often good to be able to talk to several people when one is depressed, as one needs to process experiences by talking about them on repeated occasions. Telephoning is a good way of keeping in touch.

Sometimes despondent people try to hold back their tears, but it is good to cry. Crying has a healing effect, as does laughter. Laughing is difficult when one is depressed, but for preventive purposes it is important, between bouts of depression, to allow oneself to be stimulated by books, plays, sports events, or other activities that promote good mood and laughter. An optimistic attitude towards life and a stimulating existence promote health and recovery from mental and physical illnesses.

Writing a diary, an email, or perhaps a letter, may be a good way of working through the crises associated with depression. A diary affords scope for reflection. Asking questions is an important step in the direction of steering one's own life, and daring to get out of a rut. Questions may help a person to regain a sense of coherence, purpose, and belonging, which is an important factor in health.

Try to appreciate the positive side of life, by writing a list and putting plus signs against all the good points. One may, perhaps, have a kind husband or wife, children who care, helpful neighbours or colleagues, a pleasant home, work, hobbies, a garden, or access to nature. At the end of every day, think about something enjoyable. Helping others, feeling needed, and having a task to perform is another health-promoting factor, strengthening self-esteem and enhancing fellowship.

External appearances

Despondent and depressed people usually neglect themselves and their appearance. One should attempt to dress attractively, comfortably and, where necessary, warmly. Depressed people often feel cold not only mentally but also physically. One should therefore ensure that one's home is warm enough, or take a hot shower or bath.

One can also try to repaint: warm colours provide stimulation and lighten one's mood. Rearranging the furniture may also serve as an indication that one is seeking to depart from old routines and embark on something new.

Planning enjoyable activities such as: cooking, singing in a choir, painting, sewing, playing football, building and tinkering with a car, motorcycle, or moped, are good ways of breaking the vicious circle of hopelessness. One should dare to be satisfied with personal achievements.

Diet

Regular eating habits and a balanced diet are a basic precondition for our well-being. A balanced diet contains proteins and all the important minerals and vitamins. It is good to make at least one hot meal a day, even if it is simple. Like everyone else, a depressed person should remember to eat fresh fruit, vegetables (including potatoes), rice, fish, and moderate quantities of bread, pasta, or meat. It is important to drink enough water. Slimming diets should be avoided, as they may exacerbate depression.

Tryptophan

The human body and brain need amino acids, the building-blocks for proteins. Particular attention should be paid to the elderly, whose depression may be caused by deficiencies of amino acids, vitamins, and minerals. The body itself can produce some amino acids, while it obtains others only from food. One of the latter is the amino acid known as tryptophan, which is required by the body for mood regulation. Foods containing tryptophan include: meat, milk, eggs, bananas, kiwis, apricots, plums, tomatoes, pineapples, walnuts, and sunflower seeds.

Craving for carbohydrates

Many people experience a craving for chocolate, sweets, and other carbohydrates when they are depressed. Carbohydrates are needed to provide energy and prevent tiredness, and they facilitate the absorption of tryptophan from our diet. Indulge in sweets in moderation, but exercise as well.

Exercise

Exercise is excellent for all-round health, as the increased blood flow has a favourable effect on both the mind and the body. Exercise contributes to endorphin production. Endorphins are the body's own substances that reduce the perception of pain and also help regulate mood. Walking in the woods, having a workout, skating or skiing, pottering in the garden, going for a bicycle ride, are just a few examples of taking exercise. Physical activity distracts the mind from gloomy thoughts and diverts attention from despondency. Fresh air and daylight help to curb depression.

Light

Daylight improves mood. One should take a walk in the middle of the day, when the light is strongest. Even if the sun is not shining, the retina of the eye is affected by daylight. Snow has a positive effect and counteracts depression: we feel better in the winter if there is plenty of snow to brighten up the scene. Adequate lighting at home and at work, for example, strip-lighting fixtures that emit bright white light reminiscent of daylight, is helpful.

Sleep

Sleep is vital for revitalization of the central nervous system but sleep problems are common in depression. Regularity is important regarding sleeping habits. It is a good idea to get up and go to bed at the same time every day. Slowing down and letting go of the worries that may often cause insomnia are important. One can take a short walk, listen to music, or read a book before bedtime.

Depressed people wake frequently and have difficulty in falling asleep again. Those who cannot sleep should get up, settle down in a comfortable armchair and read, listen to music, or leaf through a book they enjoy. Having a mug of hot milk can help. People who wake up in the hour before dawn, when the body temperature is lowest, should wrap a warm blanket around themselves.

Sedatives and stimulants

One should avoid drowning one's sorrows in alcohol or narcotics, as these not only exacerbate but may also trigger depression. Coffee may be beneficial, but too much may cause palpitations and insomnia. One should therefore be aware of how many cups of coffee a day have been drunk.

One must not be careless about taking medicines, regardless of whether they are for a mental or physical illness. Every change in medication and trouble-some or worrying side effects must be discussed with the doctor in charge of the treatment.

St John's wort

Indications

St John's wort (*Hypericum perforatum*) has been used as a medicinal plant for a very long time. It has become very popular in Europe as well as in the USA as a remedy against light to moderate depression and anxiety. Interest in the herb as a remedy for depression has increased in the past years, but more research is needed to provide conclusive results.

Side effects

Few side effects are noted in treatment with this herbal remedy, as it takes a while to act in the system. Ailments in the alimentary tract, such as diarrhoea, nausea, stomach ache, and loss of appetite, and also skin rashes have been reported. High doses may cause rashes and dermatitis, i.e. skin inflammation, if the recipient is exposed to strong sunlight. It is always important to consult a doctor when combining herbal and prescribed medicines.

22

Suicide and depression: when zest for life is gone

 Key points

- Suicide and attempted suicide can be prevented if help is sought.

- Suicide is more prevalent among men than among women and the risk of dying from suicide increases with age.

- Suicide is among the leading causes of death in all five continents among young people of both sexes aged 15–19.

- As treatment of depression is often successful, early detection and treatment of depression can prevent suicide.

According to World Health Organization (WHO) estimates, approximately one million people die from suicide each year and 10–20 times more attempt suicide which means one death every 20 seconds and one attempt every 1–2 seconds. This suffering can be avoided by modern suicide prevention.

It's hard, indeed, the way drops fall.
Quaking with fear, in heavy suspension,
they cling to the twig as they slowly swell—
then, weighted down, they lose the tension.
Hard to be doubting, scared, in two minds,
To sense the abyss, with its pull and call,
and yet to sit there, all of a tremble—
wanting to stay
and wanting to fall.

Translated from Karin Boye, Swedish poet (1900–41)

Suicide a global problem

The real scale of suicide is unknown, as global official statistics are available only through the WHO databank, which covers the 130 WHO member states out of the world's 193 nations (see Table 22.1). Suicide as a cause of death may be hidden under other categories and the real figures may be higher. Suicide is among the leading causes of death in all five continents among young people of both sexes aged 15–19.

Suicide affects the dead person's relatives, friends, and colleagues. In every case, immense suffering, anguish and pain follow. It takes many years for the closest family members to be able to get on with their lives, and it is usually impossible to recover entirely from such a trauma.

Depression and suicide

Depression is, the single disease that is most strongly correlated with suicide. Up to 80% of those who take their own lives have shown symptoms of depression, and many have suffered from a full-blown depressive illness. Previous suicide attempts, family history of suicide, feelings of hopelessness, loneliness, psychiatric, physical, and personality disorders are all indicators of a suicide risk. Studies show that depressed people who have committed suicide have usually not been treated for their depression.

Suicide prevention through treatment of depression

As treatment of depression is often successful, it is important at an early stage to detect and treat all depressed people, to prevent suicide. It is necessary not only to treat people in psychiatric care who have already been identified as at risk, but also to detect people with depression, in the community and among General Practitioners' patients.

Other mental illnesses and suicide

Besides depression, other examples of mental illnesses associated with suicides are alcohol and drug abuse, schizophrenia, and manic-depressive disorder. However, the mental illness alone is seldom the sole reason for the suicide or suicide attempt.

The overwhelming majority of people that live with depression, abuse, or psychoses do not take their lives. It is only when they experience a severe crisis in life or a trauma, and simultaneously lack a functioning social network and

Table 22.1 Suicide rates per 100,000 inhabitants and by country (area), all ages (most recent year available), based on WHO Mortality Database

Country (area)	Year	Males	Females
Albania	2004	5.7	3.6
Antigua and Barbuda	1995	0.0	0.0
Argentina	2005	12.7	3.4
Armenia	2006	3.9	1.0
Australia	2006	12.8	3.6
Austria	2008	23.7	7.1
Azerbaijan	2007	1.0	0.3
Bahamas	2002	1.9	0.0
Bahrain	1988	4.9	0.5
Barbados	2001	1.4	0.0
Belarus	2007	48.7	8.8
Belgium	2004	28.4	10.1
Belize	2001	13.4	1.6
Bosnia and Herzegovina	1991	20.3	3.3
Brazil (part)	2005	7.3	1.9
Bulgaria	2008	18.8	6.2
Canada	2004	17.3	5.4
Chile	2005	17.4	3.4
China (selected urban and rural areas)	2000	12.5	12.9
China: Hong Kong SAR	2007	17.6	9.5
China: Taiwan	1969	15.6	10.5
Colombia	2005	7.8	2.1
Costa Rica	2006	13.2	2.5
Croatia	2008	28.6	8.0
Cuba	2006	19.6	4.9
Cyprus	2007	3.6	0.9
Czech Republic	2008	22	4.8
Denmark	2006	17.5	6.4
Dominican Republic	2004	2.6	0.6
Ecuador	2006	9.1	4.5
Egypt	2008	0.1	0.0
El Salvador	2006	10.2	3.7
Estonia	2008	30.6	7.3

(*Continued*)

Table 22.1 Suicide rates per 100,000 inhabitants and by country (area), all ages (most recent year available), based on WHO Mortality Database (*continued*)

Country (area)	Year	Males	Females
Finland	2008	30.7	8.6
France	2007	24.7	8.5
Georgia	2001	3.4	1.1
Germany	2006	17.9	6.0
Greece	2008	5.5	1.1
Grenada	2005	9.8	1.9
Guadeloupe	1981	13.5	2.4
Guatemala	2006	3.6	1.1
Guyana	2005	33.8	11.6
Hungary	2008	40.1	10.7
Iceland	2008	16.5	7.0
India	1998	12.2	9.1
Iran	1991	0.3	0.1
Ireland	2008	14.8	4.2
Israel	2007	7.0	1.5
Italy	2007	10.0	2.8
Jamaica	1990	0.3	0.0
Japan	2008	35.1	13.5
Kazakhstan	2008	43.0	9.4
Kuwait	2002	2.5	1.4
Kyrgyzstan	2008	14.6	3.5
Latvia	2008	40.9	8.2
Lithuania	2008	58.7	10.8
Luxembourg	2006	21.4	7.5
Maldives	2005	0.7	0.0
Malta	2008	5.9	1.0
Martinique	1985	4.4	3.0
Mauritius	2008	11.8	1.9
Mexico	2006	6.8	1.3
Netherlands	2008	12.1	5.4
New Zealand	2006	18.9	6.4
Nicaragua	2005	11.1	3.3
Norway	2007	14.3	6.3

Table 22.1 Suicide rates per 100,000 inhabitants and by country (area), all ages (most recent year available), based on WHO Mortality Database (*continued*)

Country (area)	Year	Males	Females
Panama	2006	10.4	0.8
Paraguay	2004	5.5	2.7
Peru	2000	1.1	0.6
Philippines	1993	2.5	1.7
Poland	2008	26.4	4.1
Portugal	2004	17.9	5.5
Puerto Rico	2005	13.2	2.0
Republic of Korea	2006	29.6	14.1
Republic of Moldova	2008	30.1	5.6
Romania	2008	19.3	4.0
Russian Federation	2006	53.9	9.5
Saint Kitts and Nevis	1995	0.0	0.0
Saint Lucia	2002	10.4	5.0
Saint Vincent and Grenadines	2004	7.3	0.0
Sao Tome and Principe	1987	0.0	1.8
Serbia	2008	25.3	10.2
Seychelles	1987	9.1	0.0
Singapore	2006	12.9	7.7
Slovakia	2005	22.3	3.4
Slovenia	2008	32.0	8.2
Spain	2005	12.0	3.8
Sri Lanka	1991	44.6	16.8
Suriname	2005	23.9	4.8
Sweden	2007	17.6	7.1
Switzerland	2007	24.8	11.4
Syrian Arab Republic (part)	1985	0.2	0.0
Tajikistan	2004	3.4	1.7
Thailand	2002	12.0	3.8
TFYR Macedonia	2003	9.5	4.0
Trinidad and Tobago	2002	20.4	4.0
Turkmenistan	1998	13.8	3.5
Ukraine	2008	36.6	6.7
United Kingdom	2007	10.1	2.8

(*Continued*)

Table 22.1 Suicide rates per 100,000 inhabitants and by country (area), all ages (most recent year available), based on WHO Mortality Database (*continued*)

Country (area)	Year	Males	Females
United States of America	2005	17.7	4.5
Uruguay	2004	26.0	6.3
Uzbekistan	2005	7.0	2.3
Venezuela	2005	6.1	1.4
Zimbabwe	1990	10.6	5.2

SAR, special administrative region; WHO, World Health Organization.

World Health Organization, Suicide rates per 100,000 by country, year and sex can be found at http://www.who.int/mental_health/prevention/suicide_rates/en (Accessed May, 2011).

support from their family and friends, that they may resort to suicide. Suicidal people are often lonely or have problematic relationships with their family, colleagues, or fellow students. This contributes to their feeling of emptiness: and lack of involvement and purpose in life.

Why does suicide occur?

Most suicides take place when depressed people are in a stressful and chaotic life situation. The decision is seldom based on careful considerations of the value of life. Many suicidal acts are impulsive, and serve as a way of solving various conflicts in life in the absence of a workable solution. Suicidal people have often grown up in difficult circumstances and had various negative experiences they often lack the capacity to work through.

Many people who die from suicide, and most who attempt it, are in crisis. The factors precipitating the crisis vary from sudden losses such as divorce, death of a loved one, unemployment, and loss of one's home, to educational, financial, and legal problems, bankruptcy, and other forms of financial disaster. Exile, loss of identity, and injuries to self-esteem that induce a sense of shame, such as failure in a job or assignment, are examples of other factors. Prolonged and severe conflicts in the family or at the workplace and bullying or victimization are further examples of events that may contribute to people's decisions to take their own lives. Holidays, weekends, and festive times of year may be critical for depressed people who are single and suicidal, as they are reminded of their isolation.

Most suicidal people are highly ambivalent and uncertain as to whether they want to live or die. Other people's reactions may therefore often be crucial in determining whether a person is pushed further into the suicidal process, towards suicide, or whether this process can be stopped.

Suicidal individuals and the people around them

Suicidal people often tell those who are closest to them of their intentions to commit suicide. Whether the suicide process develops positively or negatively depends largely on how others react and how the suicidal person interprets others' reactions. People close to suicide may communicate their plight in a direct verbal manner, clearly expressing their intention to take their own lives by saying that suicide is the 'only way out' and that 'putting an end to it all' feels like the only solution. Sometimes, suicidal people also blame family members for the intolerable life situation in which they find themselves.

Indirect verbal suicidal communication is characterized by such statements as 'I see no point in my life' and 'I can't live like this'. Non-verbal forms of suicidal communication may be exemplified by depressed people paying debts, cleaning, and tidying up their homes, and drawing up wills as part of the process of preparing for possible suicide. Collecting different medicines or looking for means of killing oneself is another type of indirect communication.

Suicidal depressed people have a tendency to interpret everything in negative terms, and do not readily perceive or appreciate the care and concern of others. The severe emotional strain of living with a suicidal depressed person may result in family members themselves showing signs of mental imbalance or depression. It is therefore important for relatives to seek professional help to remedy their own ambivalent or aggressive feelings.

The suicidal person and the doctor/therapist

A suicidal person's emotional contact with their doctor or therapist depends on their previous experience of health care. Sometimes the doctor's or therapist's reactions may be characterized by ambivalence and irritation with the suicidal person, and this may be reminiscent of the emotions and behaviour that relatives and friends display. Suicidal people very often have difficulty in expressing their need for help in clear, verbal ways. They feel embarrassed about needing to ask for help, and although they seek medical assistance they do not always disclose their suicidal thoughts.

Suicide prevention

As suicide and attempted suicide are a major public health problem, the United Nations (UN), World Health Organization (WHO), and European Union (EU) have defined a reduction in suicide and attempted suicide as one target of their work. Suicidality and suicidal behaviour occur mostly in acute or chronic psychosocial stress, and as a symptom or result of psychiatric disorder.

In the treatment of suicidal people, both medication and psychological treatment methods is usually used. Treatment should be long-term, as the causes of the suicidal process are complex. Suicidal persons should be taught to seek help again when the suicidal impulse recurs and their ability to cope with difficulties markedly deteriorates. Repeated preventive treatment, with antidepressants and long-term treatment with psychological methods such as cognitive behavioural therapy and other forms of psychotherapy are recommended.

Suicide prevention must also focus on boosting public knowledge of suicidal behaviour, and on breaking the silence surrounding suicide-related problems. Active support for the promotion of self-esteem by teaching children and young people how to cope with life's major and minor strains, and how to support friends who feel bad and to seek support from adults when necessary is important. Work to change attitudes, disseminate knowledge, and promote health must be oriented towards whole demographic groups and carried out in sectors of society other than the health-care services—whose role in suicide prevention should be complemented with a public health approach. Restriction of availability of guns, sleeping pills, and other drugs are also important suicide preventive measures.

In *The Oxford Textbook of Suicidology and Suicide Prevention: A Global Perspective*, edited by Danuta Wasserman and Camilla Wasserman (2009), examples of successful suicide-preventive strategies and treatments are described in detail.

When the battle is lost

When the battle is lost and a family member has committed suicide, it is important for the family to seek help. Professional help may be sought both from a psychologist or doctor and from various voluntary organizations or representatives of the religious community to which one belongs. Many relatives feel, unfortunately, that the health-care services did not do enough for the person who committed suicide. These services are therefore not regarded by the survivors as the best source of support. Voluntary, non-governmental associations founded for the purpose of supporting those who have lost a close relative from suicide are therefore valuable.

Children and young people whose parents have taken, or attempted to take their lives should be assessed by a specialist in child psychiatry or child psychology, and offered crisis intervention and long-term psychological support. It is extremely important to free children from their feelings of guilt about their parent's or sibling's attempted suicide or suicide. As well as the children, the whole family should obtain professional help in working through the major trauma a suicide involves.

Recognition and treatment of depression among both young and adult survivors of suicide in the family are important and should not be neglected. Suicide and attempted suicide can be prevented if help is sought, and it is important to spread knowledge of this fact.

Index

active listening 127
adjustment disorder (prolonged stress
    reaction) 6–7, 12, 13
adolescents *see* children and adolescents
adrenaline 78, 85
affective disorders *see* mood disorders
ageing process 44
aggression 3
agoraphobia 66–7
alcohol abuse *see* substance abuse
Alzheimer's disease 44
amino acids 47, 134
anhedonia (joylessness) 12, 14, 26–7, 79
anorexia 27, 59, 60–1
anticipatory anxiety 66
anticonvulsants 102
antidepressants 99–104
    addictiveness 102
    anxiety 68, 100, 103
    children and adolescents 33
    doctor's considerations 93
    duration of treatment 102
    elderly people 44, 46, 47, 100
    family members, advice to 126, 128
    manic-depressive illness 103–4
    patient's attitude to 94–5
    phasing out 102
    and physical illness 51
    in pregnant and lactating
        women 42, 103
    premenstrual dysphoric disorder 38, 100
    premenstrual syndromes 100
    prophylactic treatment 98
    psychiatrists 93
    psychosomatic symptoms 51
    and sexuality 106

    side-effects 95, 100, 101, 102, 103, 106
    and sleep 72
    substance abusers 56, 57, 103
    suicidality 103, 144
    thyroxine deficiency 80
    see also combination treatment
anxiety 15–16, 63–8
    children and adolescents 28, 68, 73
    dysthymia 17
    elderly people 44, 46, 47
    masking of depression 51
    men 63
    neurotransmitters 78
    psychotherapy 67, 68
    sleep 73
    symptoms 64–5
    treatment 67–8, 119, 135
        antidepressants 68, 100, 103
        combination 68, 96–7
        prophylaxis 97–8
    types 65–7
    women 63, 66–7
appetite changes 12, 15
    children and adolescents 27
    winter depression 22, 23
    women 36
    see also eating disturbances
asthenia 83
attention, giving to children and
    adolescents 32
attention disorders 28
autumn depression 21, 22

behavioural therapy 61, 119
    anxiety 66, 67, 68
bereavement 5–9, 29, 45

biological endowment, stress-vulnerability model 86, 87
biological theories of depression 77–80
 brain structure and functioning 78–9
biopsychosocial model of depression 81–2
bipolar disorder *see* manic-depressive illness
body rhythms 22
 see also daily rhythm
boys 26, 60, 138
brain structure and functioning 78–9
 ageing process 44
 obsessive–compulsive disorders 67
 substance abuse 56
breastfeeding 103, 116
bright-light therapy *see* light therapy
bulimia 59, 60, 61

caffeine 73
cannabis 61, 106
carbohydrate cravings 22, 23, 134
cardiac bypass surgery 50
cardiovascular disease 7
catnaps 71–2
central nervous system, physical illness affecting 49
childbirth 39, 93
children and adolescents 25–34
 antidepressants 33
 anxiety 28, 68, 73
 appetite changes 12
 causes of depression 28–30
 comorbidity 29–30
 of depressed people 130, 144
 developmental model of depression 82–3
 diagnosis of depression 28
 diet and dieting 59–61
 disappointments 29
 dysphoria 20
 dysthymia 17
 incidence and prevalence of depression 26
 nature versus nurture debate 86–7
 pain 28
 parents and other adults, advice to 30–2
 psychiatric help 94
 psychotherapy 32–3, 96
 self-esteem 30
 sleep 27, 69

stimulation 31–2
stress 30–1, 86–7
stress-susceptibility model 86–7
suicidality 28, 33, 138, 144–5
symptoms of depression 26–8
traumatic life events 29
treatment of depression 32–3
chronic depression 12, 70
 see also dysthymia
circadian rhythm *see* daily rhythm
claustrophobia 66–7
cocaine 56, 106
cognitive-behavioural therapy (CBT) 82, 118–19, 144
 anxiety 66, 67, 68
cognitive disturbances 16, 44
cognitive model of depression 82
cognitive therapy (CT) 32, 118–19
combination treatment 68, 96–7, 116
 see also antidepressants; psychotherapy
comorbidity *see* physical illness; physical problems
compulsive behaviour
 in anorexia 60, 61
 depression concealed by 51
 treatment 100, 119
 see also obsessive–compulsive disorders
compulsive disposition 83–4, 94
concentration problems 14, 17, 28, 36, 37
constipation 15
contraceptive pills 38
cortisol 23, 85, 86
counselling 107, 121
 see also psychotherapy
couple therapy 122
crying 6, 33, 44, 127, 133
cultural attitudes 5, 51
 nature versus nurture debate 87
cyclothymic disposition 84

daily rhythm 22
death, thoughts of 14
 see also suicidality
debts 19
decision-making problems 14
deep brain stimulation 112
delusions 16, 40, 110
dementia 44
depressive neurosis *see* dysthymia
despondency, chronic *see* dysthymia

despondency, natural 3, 11, 12
  bereavement 5–7
  children and adolescents 26, 28
  diagnosing depression 12–13
  major depression 14
  maternity blues 39–40
  menopause 38
  physical illness 50, 51
  transitional phases 4
  tribulations 4–5
detoxification treatment 56, 57
developmental model of depression 82–3
diagnosing depression 12
  anhedonia 12
  in children and adolescents 28
  doctors 93
  dysthymia 17
  in elderly people 44, 45–6
  gender issues 36
  major depression 12, 14
  missed diagnoses 19
  psychosomatic symptoms 50–1
  seasonal depression 22
dialectic behavioural therapy (DBT) 119
diaries, self-help 133
diet and dieting 86, 134
  elderly people 44–5
  teenagers 60–1
dismissal from job 4
doctors 92–3
  diagnosing depression 12
  seeking help from 7
  treatment choice 93
  when to consult 92–3
  see also professional help
dopamine 56, 78–9, 86
double depression 17–18
dreams and nightmares 6, 70–1, 72
drug abuse see substance abuse
'drug holidays' 106
dry eyes 15
dry mouth 15, 57, 64, 100
dysphoria 17
dysthymia 12, 17–19
  in children and adolescents 17
  combination treatment 96–7
  gender perspective 20, 36
  with major depression 17–18
  personality types predisposed to 83–4, 117
  social phobia 67

'early birds' 23
eating disturbances 27, 59–61
  see also appetite changes
ECT see electroconvulsive therapy
elderly people 43–7
  antidepressants 44, 46, 47, 100
  causes of depression 44–5
  diagnosing depression 44, 45–6
  diet 44–5
  electroconvulsive therapy 44
  institutional care 44, 47
  relatives' role 46–7, 129
  senile dementia 44
  sleep 45, 46, 70, 71, 72
  suicidality 47
  symptoms of depression 45–6
electroconvulsive therapy (ECT) 95–6,
    110–11
  case example 111
  effect mechanism 110
  efficacy 110
  elderly people 44
  indications 95–6, 110
  patient's attitude to 96
  pregnant and lactating women 96, 110
  procedure 110
  side-effects and contra-indications 111
  sleep 72
endorphins 134
energy, lack of, see tiredness and fatigue
epilepsy 49, 110
exercise 38, 134
exploratory (interpersonal)
    psychotherapy 32, 120
eye dryness 15

family and friends 125–30
  bereavement 6, 8, 9
  children and adolescents with
      depression 26, 30–2, 33–4
  children of depressed people 130, 144
  counteracting loneliness 128
  developmental model of depression 82–3
  eating disorders 61
  elderly people 45, 46–7, 129
  practical support 128–9
  and professional help 94, 96, 126–7
  psychological support 127–8
  questioning the doctor 94
  schizophrenic patients 20

family and friends (*cont.*)
    self-help 133
    suicidality 127, 138, 142–3, 144–5
    support for oneself 129–30
    tribulations 4
family therapy 32, 122
fatigue *see* tiredness and fatigue
financial transactions 129
financial worries 46, 142
Freud, Sigmund 120
friends *see* family and friends
frontal lobes 112

gender factors 35–7
    see also boys; girls; men; women
general practitioners *see* doctors;
    professional help
generalized anxiety disorder (GAD) 63, 65
gestalt therapy 122
girls
    eating disturbances 59–61
    incidence of depression 26
    self-esteem 30
    symptoms of depression 26–8
global variations in depression 21
grief process 5–7
group therapy 122
growing 69
guilt 14, 110
    children and adolescents 26, 27
    dysthymia 18
    major depression 14, 15

hallucinations 6, 16, 40, 110
'happy pills' 95
heart attacks 7
helplessness, learned 29, 82
hippocampus 86
Hippocrates 22
hopelessness 6, 11, 16, 17, 129
hormonal causes of depression 37
    maternity blues 39–40
    and medication 42
    menopause 38–9
    postpartum psychosis 40
    premenstrual dysphoric disorder 37–8
    stress-vulnerability model 86
    see also specific hormones
hormone replacement therapy (HRT) 39
hyperactivity 20

hypochondria 46
hypomania 19, 20, 93

immune system 79, 85, 87
impotence *see* sexual disturbances
impulsive disposition 78, 79, 84
incidence of depression 26, 35, 44
inheritance of depression 28–9
insomnia *see* sleep
institutional care of elderly people 44, 47
interest in ordinary activities,
    loss of 12, 14, 26–7
interpersonal psychotherapy (IPT) 32, 120
irritability 26, 28, 37, 38, 40, 64

joylessness (anhedonia) 12, 14, 26–7, 79

lactating women see breastfeeding
learned helplessness 29, 82
libido problems *see* sexual disturbances
light 135
light therapy 112–13
    seasonal depressions 23, 96, 112–13, 135
lithium 97, 101, 103–4
    and anxiety 72
    combination treatment 97
    manic-depressive illness 20, 103–4
    pregnancy and breastfeeding 103
    prophylactic treatment 97
    and sexuality 106
    sleep 72
liver function tests 102
loneliness 8, 33, 44, 45, 128, 142

maintenance treatment 102, 106, 110
major depression 12–16
    in children and adolescents 26
    with dysthymia 17–18
    electroconvulsive therapy 95–6
    suicide 138
    symptoms 2–14
    see also melancholia
major depression with psychotic
    symptoms 16
    consulting a doctor 92
    electroconvulsive therapy 95–6, 110
mania 19–20
    characteristics 19
manic-depressive illness 14, 19–20
    anxiety 67

characteristics 19
postpartum psychosis 40
psychiatric help 93
relapse prevention 97
sleep 19
and suicide 138
treatment 20, 97, 103–4, 110, 113
masked depression (psychosomatic
symptoms) 36, 50–1
massage 122, 132
maternity blues 39–40
medication
as cause of depression 16, 45, 51
to treat depression *see* antidepressants
meditation 122, 132
melancholia 14–16
antidepressants 94, 100
consulting a doctor 92
electroconvulsive therapy 95–6, 110
sexual disturbances 15
sleep 72
see also anxiety
melatonergic antidepressants 101–2, 106
melatonin 23, 71, 72–3, 79, 112
winter depression 23, 112–13
men
antidepressants 102
anxiety 63
bereavement 8–9
despondency 3, 4
diagnosing depression 12, 36
dysthymia 20
incidence and prevalence of
depression 35
major depression 12
postpartum paternal depression 40
sexual disturbances 102, 105–7
suicide 138, 139–42
symptoms of depression 36
unemployment 3, 4
winter depression 21
menopause 4, 38–9
mid-life crises 4
monoamine oxidase (MAO)
inhibitors 100, 101
mood disorders 11–20, 55
see also specific disorders
motor activity, changes in 14, 27
mouth dryness 15, 57, 64, 100
multiple sclerosis (MS) 49

narcissistic disposition 84
nature versus nurture debate 85–7
neuroleptics 20
neurons, communication between in the
brain 78
neurotic depression *see* dysthymia
neurotransmitters 77–8, 86, 91
see also specific neurotransmitters
new mothers, depression in 39–40, 96, 110
newborn babies 40, 71
'night owls' 23
nightmares and dreams 6, 70–1, 72
non-selective monoamine reuptake
inhibitors 100
non-verbal forms of therapy 122
noradrenaline 78, 86, 101
noradrenaline reuptake inhibitors 101

obsessive–compulsive disorders 67, 68,
78, 112
oestrogen 39
osteoporosis 39

pain 49–53
antidepressants 100
children and adolescents 28
elderly people 45
reduced reactions to 110
women 36
panic attacks 36, 63, 66, 67, 119
parental home, leaving 4
Parkinson's disease 44, 49, 78, 112
persistent depression *see* dysthymia
personality disorders 83–4, 97, 138
personality types predisposed to
depression 83–4, 117
pessimistic disposition 83
phobias 66–7, 119
physical forms of therapy 122
physical illness (as cause of
depression) 49–50, 51–2
case example 51–2
children and adolescents 28, 30
direct connections with depression 49
elderly people 45
indirect connections with
depression 49–50
pain 50
psychosomatic symptoms 50–1
treatment of depression 97

physical problems (caused by
    depression) 12–14, 19
  anxiety 64
  bereavement 5–6
  children and adolescents 26–8, 51
  dysthymia 17, 18
  major depression 12–14, 15
  suicide risk in the elderly 47
  women 36
physiotherapy 122
pill, contraceptive 38
polypharmacy 102
post-traumatic stress disorder (PTSD) 66
postpartum depression (PPD) 39, 40, 120
postpartum paternal depression 40
postpartum psychosis 39, 40, 41–2
practical support from family
    members 128–9
pregnancy 39, 42, 96, 103
  antidepressants 42, 103
  electroconvulsive therapy 96, 110
  psychiatric help 93
  psychotherapy 103, 116
premenstrual complaints and tension 37–8
premenstrual dysphoric disorder 37–8, 100
premenstrual syndrome 37, 38, 100
prevalence of depression 35
professional help 92–4
  for children and adolescents 31,
      32–3, 34
  deciding whether to seek 7, 92–3, 130
  for family members 130
  patient aspects 94–8
  relapse prevention 97–8
  relatives, patients' 94, 96, 126–7
  suicide 143
  see also doctors
progesterone 39
prolactin 79
prolonged stress reaction 6–7, 12, 13
prophylactic treatment 97–8
psychiatrists 93–4
  see also professional help
psychoanalysis 120
psychodynamic theory of depression 82
psychodynamic therapy 68, 120–1
psychological theories of depression 81–3
  biopsychosocial model 81–2
  cognitive model 82
  developmental model 82–3

  learned helplessness 82
  personality types predisposed to
      depression 83–4
  psychodynamic theory 82
  social theory 82
psychosocial endowment,
    stress-susceptibility model 87
psychosocial factors in depression
  elderly people 44–5
  gender differences 36
  nature versus nurture debate 85–7
  psychological treatment methods 96,
      116–17
psychosomatic symptoms 36, 50–1
psychotherapy 93, 96, 115–23
  for alcoholics 56
  anxiety 67, 68
  changing one's therapist 122–3
  for children and adolescents 32–3, 96
  for elderly people 46–7
  family members, advice to 128
  patient's attitude to 96
  prophylactic treatment 97–8
  sexual disturbances 107
  types 117–22
  see also combination treatment
psychotic depression see major depression
    with psychotic symptoms

rapid eye movement (REM) sleep 70,
    71, 72
rational anxiety 65
relapses 12, 128
  prevention 97–8, 102, 120, 121, 122
relationship problems, in childhood and
    adolescence 28, 29
relatives see family and friends
relaxation 73, 112, 132
religious support 144
retirement 4, 45
reversible inhibitors of MAO-A
    (RIMAs) 101

saliva excretion, reduced 15, 57, 64, 100
schizophrenia 20, 67, 93, 97, 138
seasonal depressions/seasonal affective
    disorder (SAD) 21–4
  light therapy 23, 96, 112–13, 135
  melatonin 23, 112–13
  transcranial magnetic stimulation 112

women 21
see also winter depression
sedatives 68, 135
selective serotonin reuptake inhibitors
(SSRIs) 100–1
self-esteem 14, 15, 20, 27, 51, 142
self-hate 14, 27
self-help 131–6
  diet 134
  exercise 134
  external appearances 133–4
  light 135
  mind, tending the 133
  sedatives and stimulants 135
  sleep 73, 135
  St John's wort 135–6
  stress management 132
senile dementia 44
serotonin 78, 86, 100, 101
serotonin and noradrenaline reuptake
  inhibitors (SNRIs) 101
sex hormones 36
  see also specific hormones
sexual disturbances 15, 38, 102, 105–7
signal anxiety 65
sleep 12, 69–73
  antidepressants 72
  in children and adolescents 27, 69
  daily rhythm 22
  duration 71
  dysthymia 17
  elderly people 45, 46, 70, 71, 72
  growing and 69
  major depression 12, 15
  manic-depressive illness 19
  normal 69–71
  self-help measures 73, 135
  winter depression 22
  women 36, 39, 40
smoking 56, 73
snow 135
social phobia 67
social rehabilitation 97
social skills training 119, 120, 122
social theory of depression 82
St John's wort 135–6
status, loss of 4
stimulation
  children and adolescents 31–2
  lacking in elderly people 44

stress
  children and adolescents 30–1, 86–7
  gender differences 36
  nature versus nurture debate 86–7
  neurotransmitters 79
  postpartum psychosis 40
  relapse prevention 97–8
  self-help 132
  and suicide 142
stress-vulnerability model 85–6
stroke 49
substance abuse 55–7
  antidepressants 56, 57, 103
  by children and adolescents 26, 28
  by elderly people 46
  manic-depressive illness 20
  masking of depression 51
  by men 36
  premenstrual complaints and tension 37
  prophylactic treatment 97
  psychiatric help 93
  self-help advice 135
  and sexuality 106
  sleep 73
  social phobia 67
  social rehabilitation 97
  stress-susceptibility model 86
  and suicidality 138, 144
  see also eating disturbances
suicidality 14, 137–45
  antidepressants 103, 144
  anxiety 68
  children and adolescents 28, 33,
    138, 144–5
  doctor/therapist and suicidal
    patient 143
  elderly people 47
  electroconvulsive therapy 95–6
  family and friends 127, 138, 142–3,
    144–5
  global problem 138, 139–42
  lithium 104
  major depression 14
  and mental illness 138–9
  premenstrual complaints and tension 37
  prevention 138, 143–4
  psychiatric help 93
  psychotherapy 119, 138
  reasons for 142
support groups 56, 144

support networks *see* family and friends
supportive psychotherapy 121–2
synapses 78

tear excretion, reduced 15
teenagers *see* children and adolescents
therapeutic process 122–3
thyroxine 80
tiredness and fatigue 14
    children and adolescents 27
    dysthymia 17, 18
    elderly people 45
    major depression 14
    winter depression 22
    women 37, 38, 40
tobacco use 56, 73
tranquillizers 103
transcranial magnetic stimulation (TMS) 112
transitional phases 4
tribulations 4–5
tricyclic and tetracyclic antidepressants
    (TCAs) 100, 102
    side-effects 100, 101
truancy 28, 33
tryptophan 134

understanding 121, 127–8
unemployment 3, 4, 116, 142

vagus nerve stimulation 112

weight changes 12
    children and adolescents 27
    elderly people 45
    major depression 15
    winter depression 23
    women 36
winter depression 21, 22–3
    case example 23–4
    light therapy 23, 96, 112–13
    underlying mechanisms 22–3
    see also seasonal depression/seasonal
        affective disorder
women
    anxiety 63, 66–7
    bereavement 7–8
    depression specific to 37–40, 112
    despondency 3
    diagnosing depression 12, 36
    dysthymia 20
    eating disturbances 59–61
    incidence and prevalence of
        depression 35
    major depression 12
    sexual disturbances 38, 105–7
    suicide 138, 139–42
    winter depression 21, 112
work life, and gender differences 36

yoga 122, 132
young people *see* children and adolescents